SATH

D1759606

How to Do a Good Job Better
in Health and Social Care

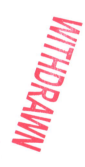

Telford Health Library
Princess Royal Hospital
01952 641222 x4440

How to Do a Good Job Better in Health and Social Care

Practical Skills and Induction Guide for Healthcare Assistants, Support Workers, Carers, Students, Parents and Guardians

E. W. Ndungu

WITHDRAWN

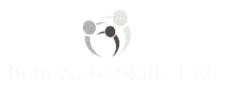

Bettercare Skills Ltd

TELFORD

CB018141

First edition published by Bettercare Skills Ltd.
133 Oxford Road, Oxford OX4 2ES, UK
Company Registration No. 8380433

Copyright (c) 2013 E. W. Ndungu

The right of E. W. Ndungu to be identified as the author of this work
has been asserted in accordance with sections 77 and 78
of the copyright designs and Patents Act 1988.

A catalogue record of this book is
available from the British Library.

First edition 2013

Condition of sale:
This book is sold subject to the condition that it shall not,
by way of trade or otherwise, be lent, sold or hired out
or otherwise circulated in any form of binding or cover
other than that in which it is published and without a similar condition
including this condition being imposed on the subsequent purchaser.

ISBN: 978-0-9576004-0-9

Printed and bound in Great Britain by
Lightning Source UK Ltd,
Chapter House, Pitfield, Kiln Farm,
Milton Keynes MK11 3LW

Note on copyright and permissions
In the case of any material that has been reproduced from a
published source, the author has made every effort to obtain
permission from the copyright holder(s); if she has unknowingly
breeched anyone's copyright she will be glad to amend the text
accordingly in subsequent reprints.

Author's note
The information provided here is for general guidance only.
All organisations have their own procedures in place.

Contents

Contents

Preface

Helping people is what drives me. However, I have realised that the best permanent valuable help I can give to people is to empower them with knowledge. Each of us has skills, experience and abilities from which other people could benefit. This book is about empowerment, which goes hand in hand with the realisation that we can do more than we are doing through acquisition of knowledge and skills and apply them to our care practice.

As you will discover, the concepts and tools you are about to learn are meant to be the start of a development process that encourages health and social care workers to continue to learn and gain qualifications that are closely linked with the National Occupational Standards for the Care Sector Level 2 and above.

In the care sector you need firm foundations. These foundations are the perceptions, attitudes, ideas, knowledge and practices you will need to embrace and act upon if you are to succeed in carrying out safe practice. Once you come to understand the basics, you will come to appreciate the difference between *doing what you want to do,* and *doing what you have to do.*

Moreover, for 'beginners' who are venturing into health and social care work for the first time, the single, greatest power leading to career fulfilment and success in any field is knowledge. Whenever we enter unfamiliar territory we experience fear and uncertainty, but knowing what to do does make a big difference. With time you gain knowledge and confidence, you handle difficult situations in a calm rewarding way for the service users and yourself. If you are not new to care work, this book should serve as a refresher and top up to your existing knowledge and skills.

To excel, learn them well, and every time a new challenge comes into your work, you need only reach into your 'toolbox' of knowledge that will empower you to succeed, empower you to provide the highest quality of care possible.

The initial stages are the most difficult and require the greatest concentration. Don't rush through the book – take your time: when you are ready to move forward, you will.

The biggest pitfall as you make your way through life is impatience. It creates stress, dissatisfaction and fear for yourself and the people you are or will be supporting.

Reading gives you an understanding but working gives you the experience when you apply the knowledge you have read. It will help you avoid trial and error in your work. When you feel you are going off course, ask for help or come back and re-read the parts that empower you to carry out safe practice.

The information, encouragement and motivation you will receive from this book, will always be here for you whenever you need it as a point of reference, because that is the foundation upon which it was written.

Finally, this book would not have been possible without the contributions of different experienced people. Therefore, I thank everyone who in one form or another assisted in its completion and success.

E.W. Ndungu
Oxford, May 2013

Acknowledgements

I am grateful to the amazing people who have supported my efforts and made it possible for me to help others. It is with deep gratitude and appreciation that I thank the following for giving both their time and their very practical insights:

To my editor Martin Noble of AESOP, who not only helped shape this manuscript but took time out of his busy schedule to make this book better and spent many nights listening to my ideas over and over again. And to those who have provided resources and guidance during the writing process: Steve Hardy, Education and Training Lead, Estia Centre; Christine Harcombe, ARC Cymru; J. Wamuhu; the staff of NHS Trust Foundation in various boroughs; NELFT, CNWL and NHS Foundation Trust; Abigail Mancin of Communication Total Oxfordshire (RNU), to name but a few; and to all those who work in this noble career.

For
Patricia
and to all of you
who are doing a good job
to help you do it better
and to those who desire to join
this noble profession.

There is always the danger that we may just do the work for the sake of the work. This is where the respect and the love and the devotion come in – that we do it to God, to Christ, and that's why we try to do it as beautifully as possible.

Mother Teresa, quoted in Malcolm Muggeridge,
Something Beautiful for God. HarperOne, 1986.

Introduction

0.1   What is good practice all about?

The principles of good practice are based on acquired knowledge and skills which will allow you to feel more confident about supporting a wide range of people in the health and social care sector to increase the quality of care.

0.2   Embedding principles of good practice

0.2.1   Who are you working with? Know your service users

Before you begin to integrate support capability information, it is vital that you understand who you are working with and what their needs are. Obviously, not all service users have the same needs. This book outlines some of the general characteristics of what are referred to as 'service user groups' in the social and healthcare sector and the baseline levels of disability awareness that tend to exist amongst them. It is important to get a clear idea of the different needs of each service user you will work with.

0.2.2   What are you planning to achieve?

Staff should primarily focus on identifying, elaborating and supporting work towards the service user's goals. If people are to be responsible for their own lives, then supporting this process means avoiding the imposition of meanings and assumptions about what matters, and instead focusing on the person's life goals.

- Have clear, realistic and relevant objectives.
- Outline the key objectives which are used to support and which are relevant to the particular service user group, e.g. communication techniques.
- Make tasks practical, fun and divide them into small sizes. Most service users have a short span of concentration, especially those on the autistic disorder spectrum.
- Make tasks relevant: it helps service users to see what is in it for them to remain involved.
- Service users' age and living circumstances have an impact on their level of receptiveness.

0.2.3   It's not just the 'what' it is the 'when' and the 'how'

- It is not just the ability to deliver support capability, it is the backdrop against which it happens.
- Even if your knowledge of support work is excellent, it must be delivered in a context that is relevant and meaningful to the service user group, the key factor, being able to engage the service user positively.

0.2.4 Work in partnership

- You cannot be all things to all people; therefore, work in partnership to access expertise. For instance: organisations that are service providers are not always experts in the field of health and social care; much of their skills, for example, lies in engaging and building relationships with professionals and specialists in that field such as psychiatrists, and Speech and Language Therapists (SALTs)
- Expertise comes through working in partnership, which allows your work to be complemented and enhanced by those who have specialist and up-to-date knowledge of health and social care issues in learning disabilities, mental and physical health.

0.2.5 Be a positive role model

Be a positive role model and positive towards service users in the following ways.

- Increasing choices – when service users choose what to do rather than have it dictated to them, they will be more likely to engage.
- Repetition proves successful in changing behaviour; the approaches of repetition often enhance learning in service users because of short concentration span and being easily distractible, especially those on the autistic disorder spectrum. Messages need to be repeated and checked for understanding before moving to the next task.
- Work with attitude and behaviour as well as offering knowledge – service users' mood can change in an instant due to ongoing factors in their lives; therefore they need to be taught the skills of communicating their needs to prevent challenging behaviour as a means of communication. They also need motivation, confidence boosting through praise and support to complete a task.
- Break activities down into small steps so that they feel a sense of achievement, even if they can only manage part of a task. Set people up to experience achievement.

0.2.6 Retain the balance

Retain the balance by:

- identifying what the individual service user needs;
- complementing rather than confusing support that the individual service user is getting elsewhere;
- maintaining staff consistency in carrying out support helps to minimise confusion;
- working within the care plan and towards the goals identified on the service user's support plans.

Finally, increasing your knowledge and confidence can have a positive impact on the people you support or will be supporting.

PART I

UNDERSTANDING THE PRINCIPLES OF CARE

1   Principles of Care

AIMS

- ➢ To introduce some basic concepts of caring and knowledge around the areas relating to working in adult social care

- ➢ To develop an understanding of a range of healthcare professions, and the values and skills required to work in a care setting

- ➢ To demonstrate an understanding of the importance of the core values in care

- ➢ To identify best practice and opportunities to achieve person-centred care in both community and care environment

- ➢ To understand the importance of respecting people's beliefs and preferences

- ➢ To understand how to support people's rights to appropriate services

1.1   Introduction

This chapter is intended to help people who are new to health and social care-work link theory to practice. It has been inserted at the beginning of the book in order to give inexperienced health and social care workers an awareness of principles of care and awareness of professions prior to beginning employment placements, to help them embed values into the daily lives and working practices of the service users. This is a major challenge, since training in values does not easily impact on practice.

The use of induction and foundation standards is part of the wider changes that are being made to the way the quality of social care services are regulated under the Care Standards Act 2000. Therefore, all new staff in health and social care sectors needs relevant and effective information and induction process to work safely and confidently in new settings.

1.2   Terms used in induction standards

Care provider	The organisation responsible for providing care services; the owner/management of the home/project
Interaction	The action and influence exerted by people on one another – how we behave has an effect on how other people respond to us
Residential setting	A 'home' set up to provide care and a place to live
Service setting	Where the social care is provided – this will affect the way that care is organised
Service users	The people being helped by the service – often this is not just the people being cared for, but also their families and friends. The

31

	term 'service users' is used because the focus is on people with a range of disabilities who are using the services
Service user groups	Broad description of groups of people cared for – for example, older people or adults with learning disabilities
Staff	This may be regular members of staff, or members of agency staff temporarily working in the organisation in a particular service setting

Note

In this book the term 'where appropriate' is used because seeking consent of service users may be difficult due to illness, disabilities or circumstances that may prevent them from becoming informed about the likely uses of their information

1.3   Principles of care and good practice

As individuals, we have choices that we can make independently, but those with learning disabilities may have that choice denied. Therefore, when choosing the right support services for someone with learning disabilities, it is necessary for support services to ensure that they are offering the best possible care and their treatment is both caring and beneficial.

1.4   The core values in care

Values are a set of principles that underpin what we think, what we do, and what we refuse to do as individuals. There are general values that influence day-to-day practice, especially in the field of learning disability social care. Some of these values and principles can be set apart as well as interwoven in ways that help create a holistic picture of good practice to better understand individual needs.

1.5   What do we mean by core values?

Core values are the values we adopt in our work, the people we support and ourselves. They are central to the way we give care and live our lives. Caring encompasses empathy and connection with other people; it is about interaction and motivating others to understand and reach their full potential.

Social care workers are expected to have basic understanding of the core values of care and what they mean in terms of day-to-day practice, which outline the foundation of the work settings through understanding the importance of promoting them at all times.

1.6   Why are core values important?

Core values are important for the following reasons:

- Without values, there are no clear guiding principles to how people will base their decision making process. When that happens, decisions are made based on what they feel is right.

- The knowledge we acquire, skills and training will help equip you to do the job, but your values and those set by Skills for Care will not only guide you in terms of how to do what you do, but will also serve to remind you of why you do what you do.
- Core values guide us – support work involves working with people who may be unsettled, disorientated, traumatised or with complex needs and disabilities. Values help to keep in perspective what is most important to us and to those we are working with.
- Core values help to maintain a sense of identity – what we hold dear to our lives contributes to who we are in the world, and so the way in which we live out our lives will be influenced by what we see as important in terms of family values, religious values, political values etc., for example those people who value animal rights may choose to live a vegetarian lifestyle.
- Core values help us maintain standards – professional values made explicit give us a framework against which standards can be judged.
- Core values help us maintain professionalism – professionalism relates to a particular set of values and workplace behaviour. A good understanding of values defines the profession of social care workers and thereby protects the service user and offers a guarantee of a degree of professional integrity. Sharing a common set of core values helps employees work together toward the same goals
- Core values help us set professional boundaries – core values helps promote and create mutually beneficial relationships between the professionals and the service user.
- Core values help promote a consistent approach to the support of service users which are beneficial and therapeutic to them.

1.7   How do we recognise core values?

The values in health and social care, for all social care workers, are set by the governing body, Skills for Care which incorporated, under its operation the General Social Care Council (GSCC) from 1 July 2012

The professional code outlines the values it upholds, and expects that all those in the profession will commit to promoting those values. The Skills for Care codes of ethics for social care workers may be found at www.skillsforcare.org.uk/gscc

1.7.1   Individuality and identity

Individuality is defined as 'the quality or character of a person or thing that distinguishes them from others of the same kind' (Merriam-Webster Dictionary). Felix Biestek explains individualization as follows:

> Individualization is the recognition and understanding of each client's unique qualities and the differential use of principals and methods in assisting each towards a better adjustment. Individualization is based upon the right of human beings to be individuals and to be treated not just as *a* human being but as *this* human being with his personal differences. (Biestek, 1961: 25)

Identity is defined as 'the fact of being who or what a person or thing is' (Merriam-Webster Dictionary). An important aspect of affording respect and dignity to people is seeing them as individuals.

- By seeing the person first and recognising their uniqueness of personality, character, abilities and skills, you begin to see them individually.
- People with disability, especially learning and mental disability, have historically been at risk of being 'congregated together' which has also led to establishing a stereotype, i.e. 'the mentally handicapped'.
- When people are labelled mentally handicapped or in other similar ways, they lose their individuality and ultimately their personal respect and dignity.
- Every service user therefore, should be recognised and respected as an individual at all times.

1.7.2　Rights

Rights are defined as 'An abstract idea of that which is due to a person or governmental body by law or tradition or nature'.

Rights are basic rules which help to promote and encourage acceptance of personal, civil, political, economic, social and cultural practices, e.g. rights to election, rights to life, and rights to freedom from torture.

- The rights of service users to take risks and to have their own decisions and choices fully respected, by enabling them to be able to contribute to society, by supporting each other and by taking on roles within – or, where appropriate, outside – their care environment.
- Recognising a person's rights is fundamental to recognising their worth.
- Rights such as education are said to be one of the main vehicles of empowerment.
- For the individual with a learning disability, the subjective experience of empowerment is about accessing those rights, choice and control, which with support can then lead to a more autonomous lifestyle.
- Legal and civil rights help to eradicate discrimination in our society.
- There are also other rights which we might consider as being important but which depend more on the goodwill and nature of people to recognise and support them, e.g.

  o the right to be treated with dignity and respect;
  o the right to see information held about us (service users);
  o the right to ensure that information held about us complies with the law;
  o the right to equality of treatment and fairness;
  o the right to advocacy and representation (independent support if we feel that we have been treated unfairly by service providers or their representative staff);
  o the right to be consulted about changes to the service;
  o the right to quiet enjoyment of our accommodation;
  o the right to reasonable privacy;
  o the right to complain.

1.7.3　Choice

Choice is defined as 'an act of selecting or making a decision when faced with two or more possibilities' (Wikipedia)

- Making choices for most people is part of everyday life, which contributes to their having control over their lives.
- Making choices is a fundamental part of our being recognised and respected as individuals; however, people with learning disabilities also have the right to participate in decisions which affect their lives where appropriate.
- Choosing to 'take it or leave it' is not a real choice as there is no option for people to choose but instead have to take or leave what is on offer.
- Choice for service users is now rightly promoted as a quality standard when care organisations advertise their services and it forms part of how they are judged.
- The vast majority of decisions by most adults with a learning disability can be tackled if the right information and options are made accessible to them in terms and language they can understand.
- Choice forms one of the major core elements of person-centred planning approaches
- Choice is therefore, an opportunity for someone to make a decision on how they want things done in their lives, e.g. service users' wishes regarding their own room decoration; clothing, everyday choices and lifestyles.

1.7.4   Privacy

Privacy may be defined as 'the claim of individuals, groups or institutions to determine when, how and to what extent information about them is communicated to others' (Westin, 1967: 7).

- Seeing a person as an individual is an important aspect of affording them respect and dignity.
- Privacy is closely linked with acknowledging the sensitivity of some personal information.
- Every person has the natural right to privacy and thereby confidentiality.
- Privacy and confidentiality require that facts or information which have been shared by someone with another party remain private and are not disclosed without the permission of the person who gave them.
- Privacy is also an act of maintaining a person's dignity when supporting them in doing things and we must endeavour to retain as much privacy and personal dignity as possible, for instance in:
    o using the toilet;
    o support with personal care – bathing and dressing;
    o knocking on a bedroom/flat door before entering.

1.7.5   Emotional needs and empathy

Empathy is the ability to understand what the client is feeling. It involves recognising and responding to other people's feelings without necessarily having those feelings. Everyone has the right to develop emotionally, and to have the opportunity to express their feelings and establish relationships. We are social beings, with 'feelings' being a natural part of our social and personality make-up; we need to feel we 'belong' and are important to someone. Feelings may not always show in appropriate or understandable ways, but they are there.

Social development is about relationships with a variety of people; it is about cooperation, being able to give and take, conflict and about participating in an ordinary life in the community. However, recognising the feelings or the emotional needs of another person requires a greater insight than just being aware of their basic physical needs. The best social care workers are those who can empathise naturally with the feelings of those receiving services and recognise the emotional dimension to whatever is taking place. Too often, service users' practical and physical care needs are addressed but the emotional dimension is not given the same consideration.

The following are examples of areas where the emotional needs of individuals with a learning disability have not always been fully recognised.

- Failure to understand that service users need to be included in funeral rites and be allowed to grieve after a death; that a period of bereavement is an important emotional and psychological process for the learning disabled as it is for other people.
- Being thought of as asexual and not acknowledged as having the same feelings and wishes to experience loving and intimate relationships.
- Developing meaningful friendships and long-term relationships could be easily dismissed as unimportant by service providers and carers alike. In some cases, where relationships exist, they have been actively discouraged or covertly controlled

1.7.6   Independence

Independence in a care user context means encouraging and supporting service users to live their lives to the full, by supporting them to make choices and informed decisions in order for them to achieve their full potential – for example, by expressing their own views on the care they receive. Care and support practices are organised in such a way as to help service users retain their independence by maximising opportunities for self-care

People have the right to maximise their full potential through physical, intellectual and emotional development, by ensuring the service user maintain contact outside of the new environment they find themselves in – for instance, home visits with their families

One of the major ways of learning and maximising independence is being allowed to take acceptable risks like travelling in public transport with support. It is nearly impossible for people to develop new skills and knowledge without taking risks, making mistakes and trying again. Allowing people to do this does not mean removing all precautions for their safety and well-being. It however, does mean recognising when we may be overprotecting people.

- Overprotection restricts a person's opportunities and development with consequent impact on their level of independence.
- Overprotection on the other hand, encourages dependence; it is important therefore, that people are encouraged by positive expectations to counteract the negative expectations and stereotypes which have been around for so long.

Independence does not necessarily mean someone doing everything for themselves. It can include the necessary support to complete an important task an individual cannot do for themselves. Independence is just as much about a lifestyle the person has 'independently' chosen, their wishes, wants, aspiration and their sexuality. A person may not be very competent with writing and numbers but it should not stop them accessing a direct payment with support.

Independence is about overall expectation and about active lives lived to the full by being included as part of their local community. The government states that the way to achieve inclusion is for people with learning disabilities to be included in an ordinary life. This includes; education, leisure and recreation, day time opportunities and, where possible, work. Social inclusion and promoting independence are the major themes of the government White Paper, *Valuing People* (2001), which sets out the strategy for future care and support for people with a learning disability

1.7.7   Dignity

Dignity is concerned with how people feel, think and behave in relation to the worth or value of themselves and others.
To treat someone with dignity is to treat them as being of worth, in a way that is respectful of them as valued individuals. In care situations, dignity may be promoted or diminished by: the physical environment; organisational culture; by the attitudes and behaviour of the nursing team and others and by the way in which care activities are carried out.
When dignity is present people feel in control, valued, confident, comfortable and able to make decisions for themselves. When dignity is absent people feel devalued, lacking control and comfort. They may lack confidence and be unable to make decisions for themselves. They may feel humiliated, embarrassed or ashamed.
Dignity applies equally to those who have capacity and to those who lack it. Everyone has equal worth as human beings and must be treated as if they are able to feel, think and behave in relation to their own worth or value. (Royal Nursing College, 2008)

The dignity and self respect of the service users is to be safeguarded and upheld at all times, regardless of;

- age, sexuality, education, ethnicity/origins, religious background or lack of it;
- disability or other circumstances, they must be treated as adult people by:

  - promoting activities that encourage service users to express themselves as individuals;
  - supporting them to overcome any shortcomings they may experience through age or disability
  - supporting them to maintain their dignity through their personal appearance and behaviour .

Disability awareness is not about political correctness. It is in part about:

- respect and dignity for the individual;
- being treated as a person first and recognising disability and their uniqueness second.

1.7.8   Respect

There is a level of respect which accords for all of us and everyone deserves to be treated with the appropriate amount of personal consideration and worth.

- Failing to give an appropriate level of respect undermines the concept of a person's human worth.
- The way people talk to or about each other and their use of language can show how much respect they afford each other.
- When we do not afford a person the opportunity of choice when appropriate or when we fail to recognise their rights, we fail to respect them as individuals.
- Respect is an act of upholding someone else's privacy, dignity and accepting their different opinions from our own – for example, respecting someone's beliefs, culture, sexuality, religious beliefs etc
- Service users must be respected, including their views and choices; the same courtesy we all expect should be afforded to those people for whom we provide care services.
- We should address people as they wish to be addressed and treat them as we would wish to be treated.

1.8   Partnership and importance of working in partnership

A partnership is a strategic alliance or relationship between two or more people. Successful partnerships are often based on trust, equality, and mutual understanding and obligations. Partnerships can be formal, where each party's roles and obligations are spelled out in a written agreement, or informal, where the roles and obligations are assumed or agreed to verbally. http://www.seasite.niu.edu/USA

Partnership in health and social care is a relationship marked with professional boundaries helping the service users take control of their lives and make decisions that affect them on daily basis through empowerment and advocacy and being able and willing to use power to empower, meet needs and resolve difficulties.

Working in partnership is a highly skilled activity requiring the ability to communicate and engage, to assess and plan, to be sensitive and observant. It is a combination of many skills, which social care workers should endeavour to acquire, and it requires a degree of humility to accept that the professionals do not have all the answers and service users have a major contribution to make to resolve the difficulties that have been identified.

Work in partnership with the service users by:

- enabling them to make informed choices and decisions about their life and actions without being prescriptive;
- understanding the meaning of prejudice and equal opportunities in relation to the service users we will be supporting / are supporting;
- recognising that service users come from diverse ethnic, cultural and religious backgrounds, and care must be sensitive, sympathetic and supportive, and carers should respond in a way which is encouraging to the service users;

- understanding that service users' lifestyles choices should be respected and not judged if different from that of staff;
- carers and staff may come from the same or different ethnic, cultural and religious backgrounds but must allow the service users choice and to respect their wishes to dictate care provision in these areas.

1.9   Aims and objectives of service providers

- To provide an environment that enables individuals with learning disabilities, to acknowledge and work towards overcoming emotional and behaviour problems, in order to maximise their potential.
- To provide an atmosphere of mutual respect between service users and staff and uphold the dignity of the individual.
- To provide a 24-hour service to service users, families and social services.
- To provide detailed care plans which are person-centred for all service users and to review and monitor these annually or as required.
- To provide a consistent and predictable approach, across a range of abilities and settings.
- To provide opportunities for meaningful activities based on individual's interests.
- To work together with service users to develop positive and alternative solutions to conflicts and problems.
- To provide appropriate support and stimulation via carefully monitored reasonable risk-taking, to enable independence.

1.10   Learning outcomes

- To identify best practice and opportunities to achieve person-centred care in both community and care environment
- Reflect on your own practice and the standards of care provided within your practice setting, and establish actions that you can take to ensure that service users are treated with dignity and respect, and receive care that is person-centred
- To demonstrate an understanding of the importance of the core values in care for the service users

1.11   Framework for reflective practice

- ➢ *Knowledge:*   What have you learnt from reading this chapter?
- ➢ *Skills:*   What do you know, or can do differently now, that you did not/could not do before reading this chapter?
- ➢ *Practices:*   How can you perform a task now better than before?

1.12   References

Bateman, N. (2000) *Advocacy Skills for Health and Social Care Professionals.* London, Jessica Kingsley.

Davies, S. *et al.* (1999) The educational preparation of staff in nursing homes: relationship with resident autonomy, *Journal of Advanced Nursing* **29**(1): 208–17.

Department for Education and Skills (2002) *Regulatory Approaches to Skill Development.* London: DfES.

Department of Health (2001) *Valuing People: A New Strategy for Learning Disability for the 21st century.* Social Care Services and the Social Perspective. London: HMSO.

Department of Health (2005) Valuing People Now – From Progress to Transformation, Department of Health, London

General Social Care Council (2002) *Codes of Practice.,* London: GSCC.

Hughes, L. (2002) The workforce for social work and social care, in L. Kendall and L. Harker (eds), *From Welfare to Wellbeing: The Future of Social Care.* London: IPPR.

Thompson, N. (2005) *Understanding Social Work: Preparing for Practice*, 2nd edn. London: Palgrave Macmillan.

Thompson, N. and Thompson, S. (2008) *The Social Work Companion*. London: Palgrave Macmillan.

Westin, A.F. (1967) *Privacy and Freedom.* New York: Atheneum.

1.13   Induction workbook

1.   Explain what each of the following terms mean in relation to the people you will be or are supporting? Give two examples of the things you can do in your-day-to-day work to promote each of these.

   (a)   Individuality and identity?

   _____

   _____

   (b)   Rights?

   _____

   _____

   (c)   Choice?

   _____

   _____

   (d)   Privacy?

   _____

   _____

   (e)   Dignity?

   _____

   _____

   (f)   Partnership?

   _____

   _____

(g)   Respect?

_____

_____

(h)   Independence?

_____

_____

2.   Write a short summary explaining why it is important to promote these values in your everyday work.

_____

_____

3.   Explain why it is important to find out the history, preferences, wishes and needs of the individual you are supporting.

_____

_____

4.   Explain the aims and objectives of service providers.

_____

_____

5.   How does your work role help the service provider achieve these aims and objectives?

_____

_____

6.   Why, in the past and generally people with learning disabilities have been prevented from taking risks?

_____

_____

7.   Describe an example where taking a risk can bring benefits to a service user

_____

_____

2   Communication

➢ To understand how to support communication for people with learning disability

➢ To understand the process of communication and recognise a range of different ways you can help make communication work

➢ To learn to recognise a range of factors which may create barriers to communication

➢ To consider ways in which these barriers may be overcome, including the use of alternative forms of communication

2.1   Introduction

Good communication is an important part of our life and central to almost everything that we do. It is always said to be an essential skill in being personally effective as part of a team at work, socially or at home.

Our ability to communicate effectively will be governed by many things but mainly on our development of skills which will help us to balance the conflicting aims, interests, rights and reactions of others with our own. Many people with learning disabilities have communication difficulties; we therefore need to think more carefully about how we communicate in our day-to-day work.

One of the main skills a health and social care worker must develop is to build on the self-awareness of their own strengths and weaknesses in communication to encourage the use of behaviour appropriate to the circumstances. Many aspects of communication come down to not *what* is said but *how* it is said.

No matter how good communication system in a setting is, barriers unfortunately can and do often occur. This may be due to environment, language or disability.

Communication does not depend on eloquence, fluency or articulation but on the emotional context in which the message is being heard. Social care workers need to know communication is key to inclusion, a two-way process and methods of communication that are most suitable need to be established. This may be speech/vocalisations or signing, or use of pictures / objects of reference, symbols, gestures, body language, eye contact and facial expressions.

Identification is an important ingredient to effective communication, unless you identify with the service users with what you are saying, and with the way you are saying it, they are not likely to receive and understand your message. Communicate with charisma, clarity, and absolute precision, people will listen more closely, express more interest, and respond to your communications in exactly the ways you want them to.

According to management gurus, *'being a good communicator is half the battle won'*.

2.2 What is communication?

Communication, as defined by most sources, is the process of conveying information from a sender to a receiver through the use of a medium or channel that is understood by the sender and receiver. While this describes communication in a very general sense, communication is far more than simply conveying information. Communication is how we exchange our thoughts, feelings or ideas; how we assign and convey meaning in an attempt to create a shared understanding; how we utilise signals or words to produce a desired effect (eHow.com)

Communication is, therefore, putting the right emphasis on and utilising all our senses in listening, seeing, hearing, understanding and then digesting the facts in a systematic manner. Only after the processing of all available information is done by the brain and the ideas are assimilated properly can we think up a proper response.

2.3 The basic functions of communication

2.3.1 Education and instruction

- Communication provides knowledge, expertise and skills for smooth functioning by people in the society through institutions of learning such as schools, colleges, home schooling and universities.
- It creates awareness and gives opportunity to people to actively participate in public life.

2.3.2 Information

- Communication provides information about our surroundings. Quality of our life would be poor without information. The more informed we are the more powerful we become.
- Information regarding wars, danger, crisis, famine, etc. is important for the safety and well being of our life.

2.3.3 Entertainment

- Communication provides endless entertainment to people through films, television, radio, drama, music, literature, comedy, games, etc. to break the routine in life and divert our attention from the busy lives we lead.

2.3.4 Discussion

- Through communication we find out reasons for varying viewpoints and impart new ideas to others.
- Through communication, debates and discussions we clarify different viewpoints on issues of interest to people.

2.3.5 Persuasion

- Communication helps in reaching for a decision on public policy so that it is helpful to govern the people.
- Communication is the means by which people relate to one another.

2.3.6   Cultural promotion

- Communication provides an opportunity for the promotion and preservation of culture and traditions across the globe.
- It makes people fulfil their creative urges.

2.3.7   Integration

- It is through communication that a large number of people across countries come to know about each other's traditions and appreciate each other's ways of life.
- It develops tolerance towards each other on individual and international levels

2.4   Purpose of communication

Why do people communicate in work settings?

2.4.1   Interpersonal skills

Interpersonal skills are those skills that enable us to interact with another person, allowing us to communicate effectively with them. They involve skills such as active listening, tone of voice, delegation, and leadership. Good communication skills are vital for those working in health and social care environment as they help:

- develop relationships to achieve healthy working relationships and to create an atmosphere of trust and honesty between service users, staff and other professionals;
- obtain and share information: communication promotes safe ways of sharing information with people using the services with other professional bodies involved with service user's care – for example, social workers, housing associations etc.;
- make relationships and promotes good communication with service users, their families, colleagues and other healthcare professionals;
- share information with people using the services, by providing and receiving information for and on their behalf;
- good communication skills promote confidence of the behaviour which plays an important role in decision when supporting service users with challenging behaviours;
- reporting and documentation by staff on the work they do with service users in accordance with the record-keeping policy of the respective services;
- people with good communication (interpersonal) skills can generally control the feelings that emerge in difficult situations and respond appropriately, instead of being overwhelmed by emotion;
- expressing thoughts and ideas; health and social care workers may need to share their thoughts about care issues or about aspects of practice with colleagues;
- effective communication skills are also needed to encourage service users to talk about what they are feeling, to say what they think or to express their needs, wishes or preferences.

2.4.2   Importance of effective communication in care environment

Effective communication and interaction play an important role in the work of all health and social care professionals. For example, care professionals need to be able to use a range of communication and interaction skills in order to:

- work inclusively with people of different ages and diverse backgrounds;
- respond appropriately to the variety of care-related problems and individual needs of people who use care services;
- enable people to feel relaxed and secure enough to talk openly;
- establish trusting relationships with colleagues and people who use care services;
- ask sensitive and difficult questions, and obtain information about matters that might be very personal and sensitive;
- obtain clear, accurate information about a person's problems, symptoms or concerns;
- give others information about care-related issues in a clear, confident and professionally competent way.

2.5   Terms used in communication

2.5.1   Receptive language

Receptive language refers to the ability to understand communication directed at you through listening, seeing or other means. It includes skills such as naming objects and people as well as following routines such as getting dressed or eating dinner.

2.5.2   Expressive language

Expressive language concerns the ability to make others understand what you are communicating, that is making one's thoughts known to others verbally, through sign language, pictures or other means. It involves skills such as organising objects or concepts into groups (categorisation) and using language in the proper social context (pragmatics).

Some people with Autistic Spectrum Disorder (ASD) (such as those with Asperger's) may initiate conversations but not respond to others' initiation, making their receptive language stronger than their expressive language.

2.6   Communication structures

2.6.1   One-to-one communication

One-to-one communication occurs when one person speaks with or writes to another individual. This also happens when a social care worker meets with a person whom they are supporting, or about whom they have health worries or personal concerns or with whom they are involved in a key working session. One-to-one communication also occurs when care professionals meet with and talk to each other or with the partners, relatives or friends of people receiving care.

Communication in one-to-one situations is most effective when both parties are relaxed and are able to take turns at talking and listening. One-one-communication:

- enables people to feel relaxed and secure enough to talk openly;
- enables people to ask sensitive and difficult questions, and obtain information about matters that might be very personal and sensitive;
- enables staff to give others information about care-related issues in a clear, confident and professionally competent way.

Good effective communicators are good at:

- beginning one-to-one interaction with a friendly, relaxed greeting;
- focusing on the goal or business of the interaction, e.g. key work session, assessing service user's needs, talking to relatives etc.;
- establishing a good rapport with service users, showing them respect, listening carefully and speaking clearly and in language they can understand which contributes to the effectiveness of the interaction;
- ending the interaction in a supportive, positive way such as thanking the person for attendance.

2.6.2   Group communication

Group communication occurs when a number of different people meet up. In a communication context, groups can have a number of benefits for participants:

- Groups tend to command more respect and have more power than an individual acting alone.
- Groups can improve decision-making and problem-solving because they draw on the knowledge and skills of a number of people.
- A group can be an effective way of sharing responsibilities.
- Groups can improve members' self-esteem, social skills and social awareness, especially where the group has a therapeutic goal.

Group communication is very common in the health and social care sector. This is largely because care professionals tend to work in teams and in partnership with service users and their families. However, groups can limit the effectiveness of communication when:

- power struggles and battles break out within the group, resulting in a loss of purpose and effectiveness;
- the group loses sight of its main goal or purpose, drifting into a pattern of ineffective activity that doesn't have a real benefit or outcome (for example, holding meetings for the sake of meetings);
- in groups people find it hard to speak and contribute effectively or to challenge aspects of the group's thinking or practices; this can lead to poorly thought-out, unquestioned decisions being made;
- the power in a group is held by a single person or is misused by a small clique of people to dominate others and pursue their own agenda.

Groups work best if there is a team leader who encourages everyone to have a say in turn, rather than everyone trying to speak at once.

2.7 Formal and informal communication

2.7.1 Formal communication

Formal communication can be defined as a presentation or written piece of information that strictly follows rules, conventions, and ceremony, and is free of colloquial expressions.

Formal communication suggests the flow of information by the lines of authority formally acknowledged in an organisation, and its members are likely to communicate with one another strictly through channels constituted in the structure. Therefore, formal communication involves a purposeful effort to influence the flow of communication so as to guarantee that information flows effortlessly, precisely and timely. It generally follows a hierarchical order.

2.7.2 Informal communication

Informal communication is a casual discussion, verbal exchange, note, or memorandum that may adhere less strictly to rules and conventions. It is communication that fall outside the formal channels and it is also known as grapevine.

- It is established around the societal affiliation of members of the organisation.
- Informal communication does not follow authority lines as in the case of formal communication.
- Informal communication is oral and may be expressed even by simple glance, sign or silence.
- Informal communication is implicit, spontaneous, multidimensional and diverse.
- It often works in group of people, i.e. when one person has some information of interest: s/he passes it on to his informal group etc.
- It acts as a valuable purpose in expressing certain information that cannot be channelled via official channels.
- It satisfies the people's desires to identify what is happening in the organisation and offers an opportunity to express dreads, worries and complaints.
- Informal communication also facilitates the amelioration of managerial decisions as more people are involved in the process of decision-making.
- Informal communication does not follow any hierarchical order.

2.8 Forms of communication

There are three main forms of communication: the written word, verbal and nonverbal. We can also use technology to communicate

2.8.1 The written word

Written communication involves any type of interaction that makes use of the written word either electronically or handwritten. Written communication requires:

- Literacy skills: The ability to be able to present the written word clearly and correctly.
- Being able to read the written word accurately. This is central to the work of any person providing a service in a health and social care environment when keeping records and in writing reports.
- Different types of communication need different styles of writing but all require literacy skills, example include letters and memos
- A more formal style of writing is needed when recording information about a service user care and progress reports.
- It would be unacceptable to use text message abbreviations, in record keeping or report writing as not all the people can understand them, such as WIIIFM – what is in it for me

2.8.2   Technological aids

These include electronic or mechanical inventions and gadgets that help people with visual/audio/speech impairment to communicate. Rapid development of technology means there are many electronic inventions that help us communicate.

- Mobile phones: used to make calls or to send text messages and emails.
- Computers: on which we record, store and communicate information very quickly and efficiently over long distances through emails or Skype.
- Communication aids: can turn small movements into written word and then into speech, such as the voice box most famously used by the scientist, Professor Stephen Hawking.

2.8.3   Verbal communication

- Verbal communication uses spoken/vocalisation of words to present ideas, thoughts, opinions and feelings.
- Good verbal communication is the ability to both explain and present ideas clearly through the spoken word, and to listen carefully to other people. This involves using a variety of approaches and styles appropriate to the audience being addressed.

2.8.4   Nonverbal communication

- This refers to communication used to express ideas, feelings and opinions without use of spoken word/talking/vocalisation. This might be through the use of body language, facial expressions, gestures, touch or contact, signs, symbols, pictures, objects of reference and other visual aids.
- It is very important to be able to recognise what a person's body language is saying; especially when, as a health and social care worker, you are dealing with people with visual/audio/speech impairment.
- It is also important to be able to understand the messages being sent with our own bodies when working with service users, other professionals and colleagues.

2.8.5   Main elements of nonverbal communication

1. Proximity
2. Body language

3. Facial expression
4. Eye contact
5. Gesture
6. Touch or contact
7. Appearance
8. Signs and symbols
9. Pictures and objects
10. Hand movement
11. Head movement
12. Posture

1. *Proximity*

Proximity means being near or close to someone or something. People often refer to their need for 'personal space', which is an important type of nonverbal communication. The amount of distance we need and the amount of space we perceive as belonging to us are influenced by a number of factors including social norms (the behavioural expectations and cues within a society or group), situational factors, personality characteristics and level of familiarity.

- People usually sit or stand so they are eye-to-eye if they are in an informal or aggressive situation.
- Sitting at an angle to each other creates a more relaxed, friendly and less formal atmosphere.

2. *Body language*

Posture is the way we sit or stand, which can send messages.

- Slouching on a chair can show a lack of interest or boredom in what is going on.
- Folded arms can suggest that you are feeling negative or defensive about a person or situation.
- Movement: the way we move can give out messages, e.g. shaking your head while someone else is talking might indicate that you disagree with them.
- Waving your arms around can indicate you are excited or agitated about something.

3. *Facial expression*

Facial expression is the movement of the face that express a person's feelings; for example, wide eyes is a show of surprise, interest in someone or recognition.

- A smile shows we are happy and a frown shows we are annoyed or disapproving of someone or a situation.

While nonverbal communication and behaviour can vary considerably between cultures, the facial expressions for happiness, sadness, anger and fear are similar throughout the world.

4. *Eye contact*

Eye contact is a meeting of the eyes between two individuals. While it is an important part of communication, it is important to remember that good eye contact does not mean staring fixedly into someone's eyes. Children and adults on the autistic disorder spectrum are known to shy from direct eye contact. Good eye contact should last between four to five seconds.

5. *Gesture*

Gestures are planned movements and signals using parts of the body like hands. They are an important way to communicate meaning without words. Common gestures include waving using hands to say hello or goodbye, pointing, or using fingers to indicate numeric amounts. Other gestures are subjective and related to culture.

6. *Touch or contact*

Touch can be used to communicate affection, familiarity, sympathy and other emotions to another person.

In normal settings, offering someone physical support through touch/contact is often seen as a humane or sympathetic way of dealing with someone's joy or distress. However, touch/contact in the work of a social care worker with service users can be seen as preventing the healing process, so alternative verbal or nonverbal communication modes can be far more effective.

In the health and social care environment, there is always a likelihood of allegations being made against social care workers because of inappropriate or misconstrued physical contact. This, however, is dependent upon the nature of services the organisation offers and the nature of service user groups using the services.

7. *Appearance*

Our choice of colour, clothing, hairstyles and other factors affecting appearance are also considered a means of nonverbal communication. Appearance can also alter physiological reactions, judgments and interpretations. Just reflect on all the subtle judgements we quickly make about someone based on his or her appearance. These first impressions are important, which is why experts suggest that job seekers dress appropriately for interviews with potential employers.

8. *Signs and symbols*

(a) Signs
There are certain common gestures made using body language, facial expressions that most people automatically recognise, for example:

- a wave of the hand can mean hello or goodbye;
- thumbs up can mean that all is well;
- using fingers can indicate numeric amounts.

(b) Symbols

A symbol is an item or image that is used to represent something that communicates information.

9. *Pictures and objects*

(a) Pictures

Picture of all forms communicate messages; an X-ray and a fractured bone can more easily communicate to a doctor someone needing a plaster and exactly what is involved. A picture of a plate and spoon will signify that it's time for food.

(b) Objects

Objects may have a particular meaning for a person (e.g. a special ring or ornament) while others may represent the same thing to lots of people, e.g. a cup may be associated with tea or coffee. Objects used as reference to something are termed 'objects of reference'.

10. *Hand movement*

There are three main uses of nonverbal communication using hand movement.

Greetings: Greetings include waves, handshakes and salutes. For example, when children see their friends in the morning on the way to school, they may wave to them.

Shaking hands: This is a formal way of greeting – for instance your colleagues at work or strangers.

The salute: This is used in the armed forces when a person of a higher rank meets his or her junior officers.

11. *Head movement*

People may use head movements to reinforce or modify what they are saying. For example, someone may nod their heads vigorously when saying 'Yes', to emphasise that they agree with another person, or shake their head to indicate that they disagree.

12. *Posture*

Posture is the way we sit or stand, and it is important as it convey messages.

- Good, straight posture indicates confidence. It tells the audience that you are in control. It conveys the message that you have confidence in your competence.
- Leaning slightly forward shows the audience you care.
- Slouching on a chair can show a lack of interest in, or boredom with, what is going on.
- Hunched shoulders indicate lack of confidence and possibly low self-esteem.

2.9   Communication cycle

Communication is about making contact with others and being understood. It involves people sending and receiving 'messages' continuously. In order to communicate you have to go through a process with another person; this process is called the communication cycle, because the process goes round in a circle. The communication cycle is as follows:

- Ideas occur: you think of a message you want to communicate, information to pass on or an idea, or to persuade someone to do something, or to entertain or inspire a service user or colleague.
- Message coded: you think about how you are going to say what you are thinking and decide in what form the communication will be, e.g. spoken word or sign language. And put it into this form in your head.
- Message sent: you send the message, for example verbally (speak) or nonverbal (sign) what you want to communicate.
- Message received: the other person senses that you are communicating; you sent a message by, for example, hearing your words or seeing your signs.
- Message decoded: the other person has to interpret what you have communicated; this is known as decoding.
- Message understood: when you have communicated clearly and the other person has understood, and there are no barriers to communication, the other person understands your ideas and show this by giving you feedback, e.g. by sending you a message back or signing a response.

2.10   Barriers to effective communication

Fixing communication problems with service users with communication deficit can make a huge difference to their lives. People can be supported better, easier working relationships between service users and staff, and easy interaction. However, there are factors that hinder effective communication;

2.10.1   Being distracted

This is influenced by the environment – too noisy, too hot, too cold etc. When we pay attention to the distracting factors we pay less attention to the conversation at hand and become distracted from the task at hand. It takes practice to block distractions and remain focused on the conversation.

2.10.2   Rehearsing your response

This happens when you are too busy and focused on preparing your response to what the other person is saying. You are therefore not fully aware of what is being said at precisely that moment.

2.10.3   Being overemotional

Allowing fear, defensiveness, anger, and resentment to take control will affect the way messages are expressed. Emotions are going to show up all the time. It is only when they overwhelm us that they become a barrier to effective communication. Communicating your message and emotions clearly is a matter of using volume, tone, pitch, melody, and pace in the right way.

2.10.4 Having an agenda

When people have a hidden agenda it is likely they will not be able to stay focused on what the other person is saying. Most likely people will be too busy thinking of how to convince others about something or of ways to ask them for something, to be actually listening to what is being said. Most people have an agenda, and one of the main reasons we communicate is to get something we want, either through control, manipulation or just influence. Having an agenda becomes a problem when people become too focused on fulfilling it; when they remain too attached to getting their way it creates a barrier to effective communication.

2.10.5 Prejudging and filtering

This involves using our personal frame of reference to process any information we get. Our frame of reference consist of ideas, conclusions, experiences, preconceptions, values and beliefs that we have about life. For example, we may disregard what someone is telling us because we dislike a trait about the person. We dismiss their input beforehand. We may reject or ignore someone's ideas because their values are different from our own.

2.11 Factors that affect communication

Barriers to communication prevent or interfere with a person's ability to send, receive or understand a message. A number of factors can affect an individual's ability to communicate effectively. These factors may include the following.

2.11.1 Sensory impairment

Sensory impairment refers to a defect in sensing and passing on the impulse. This leads to absence of sensation and neuronal coordination. People with sensory impairment may not be able to hear or speak or view or smell or feel or react to the stimuli given to the respective sensory systems. The impairment may be caused by aging and other physiological changes, disabilities, accident or injuries etc. (wiki-answers.com)

People are affected differently depending on which sense has been impaired.

2.11.2 Foreign language

A foreign language is a language indigenous to another country. It is also a language not spoken in the native country of the person referred to. (En-Wikipedia)

When someone speaks a different language or uses sign language, the person being addressed may not be able to make any sense of the information they are being given by someone trying to help them if that person does not speak their language or understand signing. This creates a barrier for information to be shared and affects effective communication

2.11.3 Jargon

Jargon is terminology used and understood by people in a particular clique, industry or area of work, e.g. doctors. When a service provider, for example a doctor uses technical language the service user may not understand. This can frustrate and intimidate the service user, particularly if they feel they are being 'blinded by science' or that their concerns aren't being responded to in an appropriate manner.

The doctor, for example, may say that the service user (patient) needs bloods tests and a CT scan. This can sound very frightening to someone who has been rushed into hospital. It is important that the doctor explains that they need to take some blood to do some simple tests and then explains what a CT scan is. Understanding the facts can make something seem less scary.

2.11.4 Slang

Slang is an informal type of language used by a particular group of people such as teenagers or buddies/mates. When a service user uses language that not everyone uses, such as saying they have a problem with their waterworks, this could refer to the plumbing system in their living environment but could also refer to going to the toilet to pass urine.

In some instances it may be appropriate to use slang with your peers but not with service users who may take the meaning literally (possibly because of an impairment of imagination). A social care worker should avoid using any language that can be misunderstood or misinterpreted or which might cause offence.

2.11.5 Dialect (accent)

People may pronounce different words for everyday objects depending on the area of a country they come from. This is because they are using a different dialect or accent. For instance, in some areas of England people say 'innit' instead of 'isn't it' and this can cause confusion.

2.11.6 Acronyms

Acronyms are the initial letters of the words in a phrase, e.g. NHS – National Health Services. If acronyms are known between communicating parties, this facilitates economy in written and oral communications, but if a person cannot work out an acronym, communication is lost.

There are many acronyms in healthcare, especially with dispensed medication and they can be confusing. A doctor might say, 'He has those tablets TDS', which means three times a day.

2.11.7 Cultural differences

Every culture has its own rules about proper behaviour which affect verbal and nonverbal communication. Ting-Toomey (1999) describes three ways in which culture interferes with effective cross-cultural understanding. First 'cognitive constraints'. These are the frames of reference or world views that provide a backdrop that all new information is compared to or inserted into.

Second are 'behaviour constraints'. Each culture has its own rules about proper behaviour which affect verbal and nonverbal communication: whether or not one looks the other person in the eye; whether one says what one means overtly or talks around the issue; how close the people stand to each other when they are talking – all of these and many more are rules of politeness which differ from culture to culture.

Ting-Toomey's third factor is emotional constraints'. Different cultures regulate the display of emotion differently. Some cultures get very emotional when they are debating an issue. They yell, they cry, they exhibit their anger, fear, frustration, and other feelings openly. Other cultures try to keep their emotions hidden, exhibiting or sharing only the 'rational' or factual aspects of the situation

In summary cultural differences affect communication when the same thing means different things in different cultures. For example, it is seen as polite and respectful to make and maintain eye contact when speaking to someone in Western culture but in other cultures, for example in Africa, it can be seen as rude and defiant. Looking down when talking to someone could be a show of respect.

2.11.8 Distress

Communication can be hindered when someone is distressed. They might find it hard to pass information; they may not concentrate on what is being said or listen properly and they could misinterpret information. They might also be tearful or have difficulty in speaking.

2.11.9 Emotional difficulties

We all experience emotional difficulties at times and become upset. When we receive some bad news and become emotionally overwhelmed, we may not hear or understand what people are saying, which can lead to misunderstandings. Emotional difficulties can be brought about by fear, mistrust or suspicion. This inhibits communication between people or in a care environment between staff and service users

2.11.10 Health issues

When people are feeling poorly, they may not be able to communicate as coherently as when they are feeling well. People may not be willing to talk as they feel uneasy about themselves, and depending on which health problem they suffer from, different things will affect their speech and understanding. This can affect colleagues and service users.

Equally, people who are being cared for in hospital because of an illness (stroke) may not be able to communicate in their normal way. Some long-term (chronic) illnesses such as Parkinson's disease, multiple sclerosis or dementia also affect an individual's ability to communicate.

2.11.11 Environmental problems

Environmental factors that affect communication and cause barriers, according to the National Centre for Audiology include:

- poor lighting
- visual factors
- noise
- distance
- echo

Communication is affected by the environment people find themselves in. For example, someone who does not see very well will struggle to read written information in a dimly lit room. Similarly an autistic person with sensory impairment may react to the environment differently: he/she may be affected by fluorescent lighting, noise or echo.

2.11.12 Misinterpretation of message

Communication is likely to be strained due to misinterpretation of messages, depending on a number of factors:

- how the message is sent;
- people's interpretation of visual cues;
- if the message is ambiguous, the receiver is especially likely to clarify it for him/herself in a way that corresponds with his/her expectation;
- if the communication is verbal, tone of voice can influence interpretation;
- given our tendency to hear what we expect to hear, it is very easy for people in conflict to misunderstand each other.

But when it comes to effective communication, the truth is that *how* you say your words matters far more than the words themselves.

2.12   Overcoming communication barriers

It is important to be able to overcome communication barriers if people are to receive the care they need. Communication difficulties can:

- isolate a person, making them feel cut off, so it is particularly important in a health and social care environment to overcome these difficulties;
- lead service users to present challenging behaviour as they feel their support needs are not being met or they are not being heard.

Barriers to communication can be minimised in the following ways.

2.12.1   Adapting the environment

This can be done in a number of ways, such as:

- improving lighting for those with sight impairments;
- reducing background noise for those with hearing impairments, and for those with autism it is necessary to create some quiet areas away from noisy activity;
- lifts can be installed with a voice prompt giving information such as when the doors are opening and closing and which floor the lift is on for those who with sight impairment;
- ramps can be added to make it easier to access buses on and off;

- reception desks can be lowered and signs put lower down on walls, so that people with physical disabilities can access the people and information they need.

2.12.2 Understanding language needs and preferences

Service providers need to understand language needs and communication preferences of the people they are providing support services to.

- They may have to reword messages so that they are in short, concise, clear sentences, and avoid slang, jargon and dialect as much as possible.
- They can explain details to people who cannot see and encourage them to touch things such as their face, use rails in building to help promote independence in accessing buildings.
- They should not shout at those who cannot hear very well, but use normal, clear speech and make sure their faces are visible for lip-reading.
- They can employ a communicator or interpreter for spoken or signed language and show pictures or written messages, depending on what is best for the service user.

2.12.3 Using individual preferred language

Most leaflets produced by public bodies such as the National Health Service (NHS) are now written in a variety of languages so that people who do not speak English can still access the information.

2.12.4 Translation

If there is a member of staff who speaks the preferred language of a service user they will help translate the message. It is always important to ask a service user what their preferred language is for written and verbal communication.

2.12.5 Timing

It is important to pick the right time to communicate important information to a service user. Speaking clearly and slowly, and repeating and, if necessary, rephrasing what you say can make communication more effective with some service users, their relatives and colleagues.

Speaking a little more slowly can help where a person has a hearing or visual impairment, a learning disability, or is anxious or confused. The pace of communication may need to be slower to give the person time to understand what is being said to them. It is also important to allow time for the person to respond. This can mean tolerating silences whilst the person thinks and works out how to reply

2.12.6 Using support services and specialist devices

Health and social care workers should understand the language needs and communication preferences of the people with whom they work. If an individual has difficulty communicating in English, or has sensory impairments or disabilities that affect their communication skills, specialist communication should be consulted. These include speech and language therapists, advocates, translators and interpreters.

2.12.7 Electronic devices

There are many electronic devices that help overcome barriers to communication. These include:

1. *Mobile phones*

   - These are generally affordable and available to the population at large, making them more accessible than computers and far more cost-effective.
   - They have many uses in health and social care. For example, they enable emergency response teams to coordinate their efforts.
   - They allow a surgical team to contact someone awaiting an organ transplant.
   - They are used to gather and send information.
   - They are especially important in health and social care in developing countries, where people may live several days' walk from the nearest doctor.

2. *Telephone amplifiers*

   - These are devices that amplify, or make louder, the ringing tone of a phone so that people who are hard of hearing and maybe using a hearing aid are able to hear the phone more clearly when it rings.
   - They also amplify the volume of the person speaking on the other end by up to 100%.
   - Flashing lights are other devices on telephones so someone who is hard of hearing can see that the phone is ringing when the light flashes.

3. *Hearing loops*

   - A hearing loop system helps deaf people who use a hearing aid or loop listener hear sounds more clearly because it reduces or cuts out background noise. At home, for example, people could use a loop to hear sound from their television.
   - People can also set up a loop with a microphone to help them hear conversations in noisy places. In the theatre, a loop can help them hear the show more clearly.
   - A hearing-impaired student can wear a loop and the teacher a microphone to help the student hear what the teacher says.

2.13 Behaviour that hinder effective communication

2.13.1 Aggression

Aggression is behaviour that is unpleasant, frightening or intimidating and frustrating. It can take any of three forms:
- physical
- mental
- verbal.

It can cause physical pain or emotional harm to those it is directed at. Aggression is caused by a range of factors, such as substance misuse, mental health, a personality problem, fear or an attempt to dominate someone else.

- Aggression is used as a form of communication especially by people with ASD.
- Aggression is a form of communication in that it communicates a person's state of mind, such as annoyance or frustration which becomes a barrier to communication.
- Aggression is often emotion that is out of control and can be destructive. When someone shouts at someone else, the other person can be afraid and will either shout back or shut the aggressive person out.
- Aggression can lead to a poorer service being offered due to breakdown in effective communication.
- If someone working in a health and social care setting is annoyed, frustrated or irritated (shouts, has a clenched jaw and/or rigid body language) the service user they are providing a service for may feel dominated, threatened and unable to respond or ask for support.

2.14 Verbal skills to overcome communication barriers

Using verbal skills effectively can help overcome barriers that might be preventing effective communication. Some of the skills needed when communicating verbally and assertively when need be with service users or colleagues include the following.

2.14.1 Assertion

Assertiveness can be described as how we recognise the rights of two parties involved. Assertion is the skill of being calm and firm in communicating information but not aggressive in the way we communicate with others. Assertion helps people to communicate their needs, feelings and thoughts in a clear confident way while taking into account the feelings of others and respecting their right to an opinion as well.

How to be assertive

- Be polite: state the nature of the problem, how it affects you, how you feel about it and what you want to happen. Make it clear that you see the other person's point of view and be prepared to compromise if it leads to what you want.
- Control your emotions: emotions such as anger or tearfulness can hinder effective communication. Therefore, be calm and authoritative in your interactions with others. You need to be clear and concise.
- Be prepared to defend your position and be able to say no. This won't cause offence if it is said firmly and calmly.
- Use questions such as, 'How can we solve this problem?' Use the 'broken record' technique where you just keep repeating your statement softly, calmly and persistently.
- Use body language that shows you are relaxed, e.g. make firm, direct eye contact with relaxed facial features and use open hand gestures.

2.14.2 Paraphrasing

Paraphrasing means repeating back something a person has just said in a different way to make sure you have understood the message. For example, if someone says, 'I have been sick since Sunday' you could respond by saying, 'You have been unwell now for four days then.'

2.14.3 Closed questions

Closed questions are questions that can be answered with either a single word or short phrase, for example, 'Do you like sprouts?' could be answered, 'No' or, 'No, I can't stand them.'

- Closed questions give facts, are easy and quick to answer and keep control of the conversation.
- Closed questions are useful as an opening question, such as 'Are you feeling better?', for testing understanding, such as, 'So you want to go on the pill?' and for bringing a conversation to an end, such as, 'So that's your final decision?'

2.14.4 Open questions

Open questions are questions that give a longer answer, for example, 'Why don't you like sprouts?' might be answered by, 'I haven't liked the taste or smell of them since I was made to eat them every time when I was a child...'

- Open questions hand control of the conversation to the person you are speaking to.
- They ask the person to think and reflect, give opinions and express their feelings.
- They are useful as a follow-up to a closed question, to find out more information, to help someone realise or face their problems and to show concern about them.

2.14.5 Clarification

Clarification means to make something clear and understandable, using a form of communication suitable for the people you are working with.

2.14.6 Summarising

Summarising means to sum up what has been said in a short, clear way.

2.15 Alternative modes of communication

Sometimes it is not possible to overcome barriers to communication, so an alternative form of communication must be found. This will include: signing, lip-reading, use of pictures/symbols, objects of reference, communication aids, gesture, body language, eye contact, facial expressions and Makaton language.

2.15.1 Sign language

Sign language is a language which instead of using sounds uses visual signs. These are made up of the shapes, positions and movement of the hands, arms or body and facial expressions to express a speaker's thoughts and feelings. Sign language is commonly used in communities which include the friends and families of deaf people as well as people who are hard of hearing themselves. Signing is a formalisation of gesture whose main features include:

- use of keyword signing;

- accompaniment to simple grammatical speech;
- used with appropriate body language and facial expression.

1. *How do we sign?*

- with our hands;
- using working hand and supporting hand;
- accurately;
- slowly and always with speech.

2. *When do we sign?*

- to attract attention;
- to answer questions – who, what, when, where, why, which and how?
- to give information;
- to check facts;
- to offer choices.

3. *The scope of signing*

- Signing is a visual form of communication, based on our natural gestures. Many signs look like the words they represent.
- There are different types of signing used with people with learning difficulties, most often used is Makaton or Sign Along.
- The signs are based on those from British Sign Language (BSL) which is the language used by the hearing impaired in the community.
- BSL is a complex language with dialectical differences, different word order and lots of finger spelling.
- Makaton and Sign Along are used alongside speech, signing the key words only in the same order as they are spoken.

4. *Why do we sign?*

- To support better comprehension.
- To encourage expressive language.
- Signing slows down the rate of speech.
- It encourages simpler language.
- It provides a visual means of communication which is easier to remember and helps those with hearing loss/difficulties.
- It provides a way to communicate for those with limited or unclear speech.
- It gives confidence to those who have limited verbal communication and relieves pressure on speech.

5. *Things to remember when signing*

- ✓ Only sign keywords.
- ✓ Remember to use speech and sign together.

✓ Make sure people can see you.
✓ Use dominant hand to make signs and other hand as base.
✓ Use signs consistently in your daily environment.

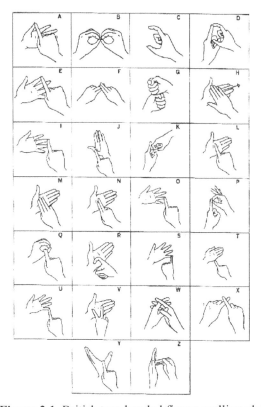

Figure 2.1 British two-handed finger spelling alphabet.

2.15.2 Makaton

- Makaton is a method of communication using signs and symbols and is often used as a communication process for those with learning difficulties.
- It was first developed in the UK in the 1970s and is now used in over 40 countries around the world.
- Unlike British Sign Language (BSL), Makaton uses speech as well as actions and symbols.
- Makaton uses picture cards and ties in facial expressions with the word to make the word more easily recognised by those with learning difficulties.

2.15.3 Lip-reading

- Lip-reading is a technique of interpreting the movements of a person's lips, face and tongue, along with information provided by any remaining hearing.
- People with normal hearing subconsciously use information from the lips and face to help understand what is being said.

- Many people misunderstand deafness, thinking that if someone cannot hear very well they are being arrogant or stupid. This can leave a deaf person feeling very isolated, excluded from everyday activities, conversations, frustrated and lacking in confidence.
- Lip-reading is used by someone who is deaf or hard of hearing.
- It is therefore important that you look directly at someone who is lip-reading and stand in a well-lit area when speaking.

2.15.4 Braille

Braille was devised in 1821 by Louis Braille, a Frenchman. The Braille system is a method that is widely used by blind people to read and write documents using a sense of touch. This uses a series of indentations made by a special stylus on one side of paper. The combinations of indentations represent letters that can be touch-read by people who understand the Braille system.

Each Braille character is made up of six dot positions, arranged in a rectangle. A dot may be raised at any of the six positions to form 64 possible combinations and these raised dots are read by touch.

2.15.5 Object of reference

Objects of reference are objects (actual) used to represent a person, activity or event.

- Over time the person learns that the object stands for that person, activity or event.
- Object of Reference are used to help a service user understand what is happening in their environment
- Object of Reference are also used to help service users make choices.

How to use objects of reference

- Before the individual starts the activity, give them the object of reference – a towel, use a sign and/or speech, for example 'now we are going to have a shower'.
- After giving the object of reference, it is important to immediately begin the activity to help the person understand the connection between the object and the activity.
- It is of paramount importance that objects are used consistently every time you carry out that activity
- Once the person has understood the connection between the objects and the activities you can use these objects to offer choices relating to other activities.
- When an activity starts, take the object of reference from the individual and put it away.
- It is a good idea to have a consistent place to keep all the objects and put them away when the activity has started.

2.15.6 Visual timetables

A visual timetable is a chart which has pictures of activities that happen from day to day.

- Some service users with autistic spectrum disorder have poor auditory processing skills and benefit from visual clues, while others who have learning disabilities may find understanding verbal instructions difficult; they may prefer to see their daily timetable in pictorial form as it aids their comprehension of the activities for the day.

- Visual timetables help a service user to know what is happening and when.
- They can also aid service users to understand that an activity has finished.

How to use a visual timetable

1. At the beginning of the day stick the activities that will take place onto the visual timetable. Go through it with the person who will be involved, pointing to each one and saying the word.
2. Perform the first activity on the visual timetable.
3. When the activity is finished, take the picture off the visual timetable. Make sure the person who has been doing the activity is involved in this, as it will help them understand that the activity is finished.
4. Show the individual the next activity on the visual timetable. Carry out the activity and together remove the picture and put them away to signify the end of that activity.

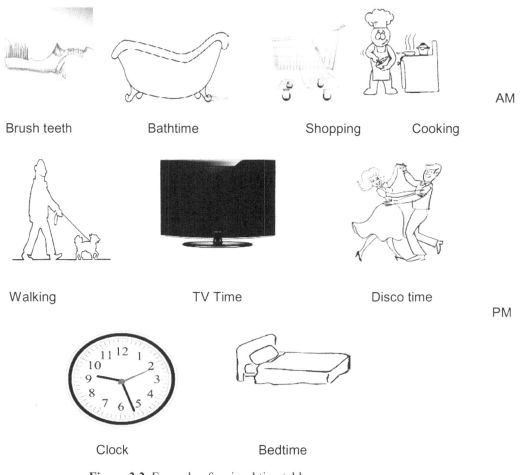

Brush teeth   Bathtime   Shopping   Cooking   AM

Walking   TV Time   Disco time

PM

Clock   Bedtime

Figure 2.2 Example of a visual timetable.

2.15.7 Social stories

Social stories were designed by Carol Gray (Gray and McAndrew, 2001), based on the idea of reinforcing appropriate behaviour. They are short, written stories to help the service user understand a small part of their social world and behave appropriately within it

Importance of social stories as a communication tool

- Each social story provides clear, concise and accurate information about what is happening in a specific social situation, outlining why it is happening and what a typical response might be in that social situation.
- Each social story aims to provide answers to key questions about a social situation that is problematic to the service user.
- An effective social story can enable a person to revisit the same social situation regularly, and remind them of their personal role in that social situation.
- Social stories are equally beneficial to staff because they learn to deal and alter the way they deal with difficult social situations and help staff develop more awareness that they are often a part of the problem not just the answer.

2.15.8 Communication passport (www.communicationpassport.co.uk)

- Communication passports are a practical and person-centred way of supporting children, young people and adults with disabilities who may find it difficult to communicate with speech.
- They are a clever way of putting complex information together and presenting it in an easy-to-follow format.
- They are easy to read, informative, useful and fun and have been widely used throughout the UK and Europe for children and adults who cannot easily communicate, or speak for themselves.

1. *Features of the communication passport*

- Communication passports have information about how a person communicates – verbal or nonverbal.
- It contains information of what the person's likes and dislikes are.
- Communication passports are used as an introduction to the person and as a way of helping to start conversations.

2. *How to use the communication passport*

- The person should have the communication passport with them at all times, attached to their wheelchair or in their bag so that it is easily accessible.
- Whenever a service user meets a new person s/he gets out the communication passport and looks at it with the new person. S/he can use it to introduce themselves or the new person can read it with him/her.
- Communication passport can also be looked at by people who have already met the service user as a reminder of how best to interact with him/her.

3. *How to make a communication passport*

In order to make a practical personal-centred communication passport the person for whom it is made should be involved. Remember to keep it fairly short. It can be made up into different forms that can help communicate this information, e.g. A3-size booklet, DVD or box of objects.

(a)   Select the person who wants to tell others about themselves

(b)   With the person make a list of things that would be useful for others to know in order to offer help and support, such as:

- the person's names and where they live;
- how the person communicates and how to communicate with them;
- things that the person likes and does not like;
- places the person likes to visit;
- any medical condition, e.g. epilepsy, what medication they take and how to support them in case of a fit.

2.15.8   Personal communication dictionary / personal gesture dictionary

According to Doyle and Doyle Iland (2004), 'a Communication Dictionary is a method of writing down and sharing information that has been learned about what the individual says or does, what it usually means and how the individual expects others to respond.'

A personal communication dictionary (PCD) helps to outline the ways in which an individual communicates. This is important for people who don't communicate using methods such as speech, writing or symbols. For people who have complex communication needs, it is important that their communication partners recognise and understand their communication behaviours.

A personal communication or personal gesture dictionary (PGD) contains individual communicative signals, what they mean and how the individual expect other people to respond. This can help to ensure all staff are aware of the individual's communication behaviours and agree on how to respond.

It assists primary communication partners to respond in a predictable manner to the individual so that an individual's communication method is being understood and responded to appropriately.

The information on the PCD should serve as a guide and provide ideas that help everyone respond more consistently and respectively to the individual improving and meeting the individual's wishes and preferences

How to create a personal communication / personal gesture dictionary

- It should have the person's name, date it was created and by whom.
- It should be kept where it is easily accessible by all new members of staff and carers supporting the individual.

To create a PCD/PGD, people who know the individual well, such as family members and those who knew him from the past, should contribute information, from their observation and descriptions of the person's behaviours, determine what these behaviours mean and then agree on an appropriate response.

Why review and update a PCD/PGD?

Personal communication/gesture dictionaries need to be regularly reviewed and updated continuously as the individual grows and learns and as others discover more about how the individual communicates. Communication behaviours can change as the individual pick up new behaviours and learn new signs. Sometimes one communication signal can have more than one meaning.

Table 2.1   Sample personal communication dictionary

Written with help of mum Diane, carers Jane and Jenny Kimanis, speech and language therapist (SALT)		
January 2006		
What I do....	What it might mean.....	What should you do.......?
Banging the side of the bed in the morning	I am awake	Help me get out of bed
Touching the centre of my left hand with my right hand hunched fingers together	I want something to eat. Please give me breakfast- toast and a drink	I will walk to the fridge and will point what I want. please support me to get it/ or toast it e.g. put slice of bread in toaster
Run my fingers of my right hand on the fore arm of my left hand	I'd like to go for a walk	Take me out for a walk
Fold my right hand and stick the elbow out	I'd like to go for a drive (seen from how his dad put his arm on the car window while driving)	Tell me when we are going out for a drive.
Touching my chin with my forefingers	I am asking for dinner when will it be ready?	Inform me when to expect it, like for instance after the drive or after an activity
Spreading my curved hands over each ear	Can I listen to music with my headphones	Direct me to my music and support to me put the CD/tape on

2.16   Communication aids

A communication aid helps a person to communicate more effectively with those around them. These aids range from simple letters boards to sophisticated piece of computer equipment.

2.16.1 Technological aids

- Mobile phones are be used to make calls but we can also use them to send text messages and emails
- Computers are used to record, store and communicate information very quickly and efficiently over long distances.
- The voice box was most famously used by the scientist, Professor Stephen Hawking. It can turn small movements into the written word and then into speech.

2.16.2 Telephone amplifiers

These are devices that amplify, or make louder, the ringing tone of a phone so that people who are hard of hearing and maybe using a hearing aid can hear the phone more clearly. An amplifier amplifies the volume of the person speaking on the other end by up to 100%.

Flashing lights are other devices attached on telephones so that someone who is hard of hearing can see that the phone is ringing when the lights flash.

2.16.3 Hearing loops

- A hearing loop system helps people with hearing difficulties who use hearing aids or loop listeners hear sounds more clearly because it reduces or cuts out background noise.
- You can also set up a loop with a microphone to help hear conversations in noisy places such as in the theatre.
- A hearing impaired student can wear a loop and the teacher a microphone to help the student hear what the teacher says.

2.17 Human aids in communication

Human aids are people who help others communicate with each other. These include the following.

2.17.1 Interpreters

Interpreters are people who communicate information, whether it be spoken or signed, to someone in a different language they will understand. This is not easy because they not only have to interpret the words or signs but they also have to find a way of expressing the meaning of the words clearly.

2.17.2 Translators

Translators are people who translate from one language into another; they communicate recorded information, such as the written word or spoken word from one language into another language as professionals. They convey the meaning as well as the message.

2.17.3 Signers

Signers are people who can communicate using a sign language, Makaton or Sign Along or using the British Sign Language (BSL) They use non-manual behaviours to show emotion, emphasise a point, make a negative statement, and ask questions.

2.17.4 Speech and language services

This service can support people who have communication difficulties and have problems with their speech. These include language and speech therapist and psychologists.

2.17.5 Advocacy services

This service can support people who are unable to speak up for themselves. This service tries to understand the needs, wishes and preferences of people, and will argue on their behalf. For example people suffering mental health who have no capacity, service users with speech and auditory impairment in care environment or those receiving care in their own home.

2.18 Good practice of effective communication

Effective communication is a process where a message is received and understood by the receiver in the manner that the sender intended it to be, through active listening, body language, facial expressions and eye contact.

2.18.1 Active listening and body language

Listening to people involves more than just hearing what they are saying. To listen well you need:

- to be able to hear the words being spoken, thinking about what they mean, then thinking what to say back to the person;
- to show that you are listening and that you are thinking about what is being said by your body language, facial expressions and eye contact.

Signs of absence of active listening

- To yawn or looking at your notes when someone is talking to you gives the impression of being bored by what is being said.
- To shake your head and frowning are signs showing that you disagree with, or disapprove of, what the person is saying.

The process of active listening involves:

- allowing the person talking time to explain without interrupting;
- giving encouragement by smiling, nodding and making encouraging remarks such as, 'That's interesting' and 'Really?'
- asking questions for clarification, such as, 'Can you explain that again please?'
- showing empathy by making comments such as, 'That must be making life really hard for you';
- looking interested by maintaining eye contact and not looking at your watch every three minutes;
- not being distracted by anything, such as a ringing mobile – switch it off or put it on silence;

- summarising to check that you have understood the other person; you can do this by paraphrasing, 'So what you mean is …?'

2.18.2 Use of appropriate language

Use of appropriate language is important and people adjust how they speak depending on who they are with and who is listening to them.

- Things that are said with a group of friends or at a family gathering might not be understood by others because we use different types of language in different situations. (formal/informal communication).
- People unconsciously change their use of dialect depending on who they are speaking to.
- A person's accent or dialect may become more pronounced when they are speaking to someone from their family or from the same area they grew up in.

2.18.3 Tone of voice

When you talk to someone in a loud voice with a fixed tone the person you are speaking to will think you are angry with them. On the other hand, when you speak calmly and quietly with a varying tone, the other person will think you are being friendly and kind. Therefore it is important to remember that it is not just what you say, but also the way in which you say it, that matters in communicating your information.

2.18.4 Pace

When you speak really quickly and excitedly, the person listening to you will not be able to hear everything you say. When you keep hesitating or saying 'um' or 'er' it makes it harder for people to concentrate on what you are saying. However when you speak at a steady pace, you will be able to deliver your message more clearly and the other person will be able to hear every word you say.

2.18.5 Proximity

Proximity is the physical space between people during interactions.

- In a formal situation, such as a doctor talking to a patient, the doctor does not sit too close to the patient in order not to invade their personal space.
- In an informal situation, people who are friends or intimate with each other will often sit closer to each other.
- People usually sit or stand so they are eye-to-eye if they are in an informal or aggressive situation.
- Sitting at an angle to each other creates a more relaxed, friendly and less formal atmosphere.

2.19 Skills for effective communication

- When you have not heard, or read, and understood a message properly it is impossible to make the best use of the information.

- When someone has communicated a need or an issue to you, then your main priority should be to support him or her in meeting it.
- Following up on an issue is the only way to convince others with whom you need to communicate that you have listened to them and that their problems or issues are important to you as well.

2.19.1 Improving body language skills

Body language is a form of nonverbal communication, which consists of body posture, gestures, facial expressions, and eye movements. Humans send and interpret such signals almost entirely unconsciously.

- The use and proper understanding of body language for communication is naturally an important part of improving communication skills.
- The understanding of body language is necessary in order to recognise the underlying sentiment which makes the person 'say' what s/he is saying, and then see if their body language is conflicting against their spoken word.

2.19.2 Improving verbal and written communication skills

Written communication can be defined as any type of interaction that makes use of the written word. It is one of the two main types of communication, along with oral/spoken communication.
It has three main elements; structure (the way the material is laid out), style (the way the material is written) and content (what the material written is about).

- Health and social care workers need to be able to communicate well with the written word. This could be by writing reports and record-keeping, such as a letter to refer a service user to a different service, a record of a person's condition and support needs or entitlement to a benefit.
- Health and social care workers need to be able to use different ways of presenting information, such as letters, memoranda, emails, reports or filling forms. When writing they should make their meaning absolutely clear (content) and structure the information well and in an appropriate manner (style). That is, to use grammar, spelling and punctuation correctly.
- Writing should be legible so that the person the information is intended for can actually read and understand it, and the language used is appropriate.
- Healthcare professionals should not use lots of technical words, acronyms or jargon when they are writing to someone who is not in their professional as they will not be understood.
- For effective partnership health and social care workers should read information provided by other healthcare professionals thoroughly, be able to identify the main points and be able to find other information from a wide variety of sources – for example electronically and on the Internet.
- Health and social care workers also need information technology (IT) skills to update records and to access information electronically on the computer or on the Internet.

2.19.3 How to develop good communication skills in a care setting

1. *Reach a common ground*

Developing perfect communication is possible especially in delicate situations through a good and a positive approach, such as talking cordially to service users about what they like and dislike and avoiding sensitive issues depending on timing and being tactical.

2. *Don't be ethnocentric*

Being 'ethnocentric' means considering one's culture as 'always right' whereas anything that doesn't conform to one's culture is 'always wrong'. We live in a global society, and this translates into the possibility of dealing with service users and co-workers with values much different from the ones we have. Devaluating somebody else's cultural heritage and considering it inherently wrong is setting up a communication barrier.

3. *Understand the world of this person and accept its uniqueness*

- Communication is understanding, which means respecting someone's tastes about, for instance, music or food, religious beliefs, culture, sexuality, choices and the decisions they make.
- Try to experience something from the service user's world – for example a person who is autistic may find too much information hard to process within their immediate environment and this can lead to anxiety

4. *If a service user doesn't respond to your efforts, do not insist*

It takes two people (or more) to communicate – you cannot do it alone. When a service user is non-communicative, avoid talking until s/he reconsiders and decides to talk to you. Insisting on talking will only make both sides angry and frustrated

2.20 Learning outcomes

- Know the different forms of communication – verbal and nonverbal.
- Understand the need to support communication for people with learning disability.
- Recognise a range of different ways you can help to make communication work.
- Understand barriers to effective communication and recognise when communication is not working and ways to make it work.
- It is vital to communicate effectively and to understand how communication is central to the services provided.

2.21 Framework for reflective practice

- ➢ *Knowledge*:   What have you learnt from reading this chapter?
- ➢ *Skills:*   What do you know, or can do differently now, that you did not/could not do before reading this chapter?
- ➢ *Practices:*   How can you perform a task now better than before?

2.22   References

Allen, B.J. (2004) *Difference Matters: Communicating Social Identity.* Long Grove, IL: Waveland Press.

Chant S, Jenkinson T, Randle J, and Russell G (2002) Communication skills: some problems in nursing education and practice. *Journal of Clinical Nursing* **11**(1): 12–21.

Doyle, B.T. and Doyle Iland, E. (2004) *Autism Spectrum Disorders from A to Z: Assessment, Diagnosis and More.* Arlington, TX: Future Horizons.

Goldbart, J. and Caton, S. (2010) *Some Good Ways to Communicate with People with Very Complex Needs.* London: Mencap.

Gray, C. and McAndrew, S. (2001) *My Social Stories Book.* London: Jessica Kingsley Publishers.

Hardy, C. (2000) *Information and Communications Technology for All.* London: David Fulton.

Hargie, O. (2006) *The Handbook of Communication Skills.* London: Routledge.

Kelly, A. (1996) *A Social Communication Skills Package.* Bicester: Winslow.

Ley, P. (1988) *Communicating with Patients: Improving Communication, Satisfaction and Compliance.* London: Croom Helm.

McLeod, S.A. (2008) *Person Centred Therapy.* Retrieved from http://www.simplypsychology.org/client-centred-therapy.html

Nind, M. and Hewett, D. (1994) *Access to Communication: Developing the Basics of Communication with People with Severe Learning Difficulties through Intensive Interaction.* London: David Fulton.

Park, E.K. and Song, M. (2004) Communication barriers perceived by older patients and nurses *International Journal of Nursing Studies* **42**: 159–66.

Shore, S. and Rastelli, L.G. (2006) *Understanding Autism for Dummies.* New York: John Wiley & Sons, Inc.

Silverman, J., Kurtz, S.M. and Draper, J. (2005) *Skills for Communicating with Patients*, 2nd edn. Oxford: Radcliffe Publishing.

Thompson, N. (2002) *People Skills*, 2nd edn. London: Palgrave Macmillan.

Thompson, N. (2003) *Communication and Language: A Handbook of Theory and Practice.* London: Palgrave Macmillan.

Thompson, N. and Thompson, S. (2008) *The Social Work Companion.* London: Palgrave Macmillan.

Ting-Toomey, S. (1999) *Communicating across Cultures.* New York: Guilford Press.

Wendt, J. (1984) D.I.E.: A way to improve communication. *Communication Education* **33**: 397–401.

2.23   Induction workbook

1. Give four reasons why people communicate.

    _____

    _____

2. Identify four barriers of communication and how to reduce or overcome them.

    _____

    _____

3. Identify four methods to encourage communication.

    _____

    _____

4. Explain why behaviour may be an important form of communication for people with learning disabilities/difficulties.

    _____
    _____

5. What do you understand by the terms verbal and nonverbal communication.

    _____
    _____

6. Identify eight aspects of nonverbal communication. Nonverbal communication includes:

    (a)   Body language
    (b)   _____
    (c)   _____
    (d)   _____
    (e)   _____
    (f)   _____
    (g)   _____
    (h)   _____

7. Explain and list five skills you can use to promote communication.

    _____
    _____

8. Explain how appropriate touch can promote communication.

    _____
    _____

9. What types of touch would never be appropriate?
    Identify three situations when the use of touch would not be appropriate;

    _____
    _____

10. Describe and identify alternative mode of communication you can use to support an individual with learning disability.

    _____
    _____

11. Explain why it is important to reflect on your work activities.

    _____
    _____

3 Confidentiality

AIMS

➢ To be able to explain confidentiality in the workplace

➢ To be able to put the knowledge of confidentiality to everyday work practice

➢ To ensure the confidentiality of service users is adhered to as per organisations policies and procedures

➢ To be able to relate to any organisation's policies on confidentiality to legislation and law

3.1 What is confidentiality?

Confidentiality is the preservation of secret information concerning the client which is disclosed in the professional relationship. Confidentiality is based on a basic right of the client; it is an ethical obligation of the caseworker and is necessary for the effective casework service. The client's rights, however, is not absolute. Moreover, the client's secret is often shared with other professional persons within the agency and in other agencies; the obligation then binds all equally.

(Biestek (1961) quoted in Thomson (2000).

Confidentiality is crucial in enabling a service user to feel comfortable enough to discuss sensitive personal matters. It is important that they feel that they are able to speak openly without the information they provide being widely available and that health and social care professional are trustworthy.

3.2 The right to confidentiality

In establishing and maintaining a positive relationship with service users to promote their well-being, the right to confidentiality is linked to the right of privacy, as confidentiality involves privacy of information.

As health and social care professionals, social care workers need to be aware that they have access to personal sensitive information about service users. It is their responsibility that they pass on only information to those entitled to receive it, on a need-to-know basis.

3.3 Why there can never be complete confidentiality

There can never be complete confidentiality. Whilst the Data Protection Act (1998) allows the sharing of information within an organisation, the information must still be handled appropriately and not disclosed carelessly to those without legitimate need to know. The information will be shared:

- between professional workers in care organisations to ensure good quality care, e.g. social workers, speech and language therapist etc.
- with managers to ensure accountability and to enable standards to be monitored.

- when written records for the benefit of the team are carried out, such as communication book, contact sheets, log books. However, these should contain general information only.

It is expected that staff within a team will share personal information on service users to enable them to manage and deliver a service effectively. This process will include relief and agency staff engaged at the service. Personal information should be referenced to specific entries in service users' daily diaries, personal files rather than openly recorded, e.g. in the communication book.

3.4 Elements of good practice

- Avoid passing on confidential information during informal conversations on service users or colleagues.
- Write up records in a way that keeps all service users' information confidential from each other. If you have to refer to another service user in another's daily notes remember to use initials.
- Never promise to keep a secret (remember, it may put someone at risk). It is important to remind the service users that should there be a situation of risk, you (the care worker) will have to share the information with the service manager. If significant information is not passed on to a service manager or team leader, there may be several risks:

  o The care worker may find themselves compromised.
  o There may be a failure to meet the service user's needs because others are unable to take the necessary action.
  o The service user may be at risk as secrets may lead to an inappropriate relationship.
  o Other people may be at risk because the information was not shared.

- Service users should, where appropriate, be asked to give consent if information is to be shared.
- Files or records should be stored in a safe place and not removed from the offices where they are kept.

The following elements of good practice should apply to sharing information of personal nature without consent outside of the team environment in order to:

1. facilitate the delivery of corporate services, e.g. income recovery;
2. ensure consistency in support, progression and recovery when a service user transfers between services;
3. enable effective internal audit and evidence of care being given;
4. reduce the potential risk to health, safety and well-being of service users and staff;
5. for monitoring and review purposes.

3.5 Consent to disclosure

All service users must be encouraged to sign a confidentiality agreement where appropriate, which must be kept on their personal file. This confidentiality agreement sets out:

- what information will be processed and kept on record about them by the service providers;
- what information will be shared;
- under what circumstances information will be disclosed;
- what the information will be used for.

All information passed between the organisation and other agencies should be set out in the agreement with the service user where appropriate so that service users understand what information is held about them, with whom it will be shared, and under what circumstances. Their permission should be sought before sensitive information is passed to others. Wherever possible they should be able to control disclosure about themselves.

Health and social care professionals should only seek information about service users on a need-to-know basis. The service user should understand what information can be disclosed without their consent.

3.6 Breaking confidentiality

Personal information can only be shared with statutory agencies without the consent of the service user:

1. to comply with the law in the prevention or detection of crime or fraud in connection with legal proceedings (e.g. request from the police);
2. where disclosure involves a child or vulnerable adult protection issue;
3. where there is a clear health and safety risk – for instance, where withholding information might cause a risk to the health and safety of staff, members of the general public or where there is a possibility of self-neglect or serious deterioration in the health or well-being of a service user;
4. for tax purpose required by law – HMRC/council tax registration;
5. in circumstances where very sensitive information may have to be disclosed – even in the face of a refusal by the service user; this happens where there is a likelihood of harm if the information is not disclosed. For example, a general practitioner (GP) has a patient suffering from a serious mental disorder in need of hospital treatment but refusing it; the GP should provide the information to the relevant authorities for them to determine if the service user needs detainment under the Mental Health Act (1983) for treatment.

3.7 Confidentiality policy

3.7.1 Primary aim

The primary aim of confidentiality policy is to protect and promote personal information and the right to confidentiality and privacy of individual service users, staff members, volunteers and others with regard to processing and disclosure of personal information.

This policy applies to all personal information held by an organisation in respect to Board and Committee members, staff, people on placements, volunteers, contractors, service users, potential service users, and applicants for employment, landlords and others.

Personal information is data relating to an individual from whom they can be identified, e.g. name, address, tax details or national insurance number, ethnic origin, health status, income support needs, tenancy history etc, which is held on file, electronically and /or in hard copy. Processing this information is subject to the Data Protection Act 1998.

3.7.2   Secondary aim

The secondary aim of confidentiality and privacy policy is to protect commercially sensitive information from unauthorised possession or use.

Commercially sensitive information is non-personal information about the organisation, its objectives or activities, which is intended solely for internal use because its release could give unfair advantage to external organisations and competitors. However this information is not protected under the Data Protection Act 1998.

3.8   Confidentiality and legislation

Organisations must have due regard to the law in protecting the rights of individuals – primarily the Data Protection Act 1998, the Human Rights Act 1998 (Article 8), Public Interest Disclosure Act 1998, Crime and Disorder Act 1998, Local Government Act 2000, and Social Security Fraud Act 2001, as amended.

3.8.1   The Data Protection Act 1998 *(www.legislation.org.uk/)*

- The Data Protection Act (1998) is the legislation that provides a framework that governs the processing of information that identifies living individuals – personal data in data protection terms, e.g. name, physical address, tax details, ethnic origin etc.
- The processing of data includes holding, obtaining, recording, using and disclosing of information and the Act applies to all forms of media, including paper and images.
- It applies to confidential patient information but is far wider in its scope, in that it also covers staff records.

The Act identifies eight data protection principles that set out standards for information handling and set the foundations for personal data to be:

1. processed fairly and lawfully;
2. processed for specified purposes;
3. adequate, relevant and not excessive;
4. accurate and kept up to date;
5. not kept for longer than necessary;
6. processed in accordance with the rights of data subjects;
7. protected by appropriate security (practical and organisational);
8. not transferred outside the EEA without adequate protection.

3.8.2   Human Rights Act 1998

Article 8 of the Human Rights Act (1998) establishes a right to 'respect for private and family life'. This underscores the duty to protect the privacy of individuals and preserve the confidentiality of their health records. Current understanding is that compliance with the Data Protection Act (1998) and the common law of confidentiality should satisfy human rights requirements. There is also a more general requirement that actions that interfere with the right to respect for private and family life (e.g. disclosing confidential information) must also be justified as being necessary to support legitimate aims and be proportionate to the need.

3.8.3   Access to Health Records Act 1990

The records of deceased people are protected by the provisions of the Access to Health Records Act (1990). These apply only to health records created after 1 November 1991. Where a patient has died, records created after the said date may only be accessed by:

- the legal personal representative of the deceased (i.e. the executor of the deceased's will or [where there is no will] the administrator of his/her estate);
- a person with a possible claim arising out of the death of the patient. It may, for example be an insurance claim. In this case the person is entitled only to such information as is relevant to the potential claim. It should be noted that if the deceased patient gave a written instruction that any of the above were not to see his/her records, such an instruction overrides the rights contained in the 1990 Act and must be respected. There are no rights of access to records created before 1 November 1990 and the usual rules of confidentiality apply.

3.8.4   Administrative law

Administrative law governs the actions of public authorities. According to well-established rules, a public authority must possess the power to carry out what it intends to do. If not, its action is *ultra vires*, i.e. beyond its lawful powers.

3.8.5   Organisations' responsibilities

In order to protect the confidentiality and privacy of service users, organisations should require by means of a contract or written agreement, any individual or organisations delivering services on its behalf to:

- comply with the law regarding the protection and disclosure of personal information;
- not to disclose personal information without a prior written consent of the persons concerned;
- not to attempt to gain personal or commercially sensitive information they are not authorised to have;
- keep personal and commercially sensitive information securely whilst in their possession.

3.9   Rights to access

The Data Protection Act 1998 gives service users:

- rights to access their manual held data and records; this must be considered at all times when staff are undertaking records and documentation;

- legal rights of access to their computer/electronic held records and all other information held on them subject to access;

• All service users' records can be required as evidence in a court of law, professional conduct committee and other similar regulatory bodies. Service users can make correction on any incorrect or misleading information and can seek compensation if any personal information is misused.

3.10   Confidentiality and record-keeping

1. Information contained in service users records should be held in complete confidence and viewed only by those directly involved in the care of the service users or authorised personnel.
2. The service user can give written consent for release of information to specified individuals. While particular services have their own confidentiality policies, consent from the service user may be sought prior to release of information to other professionals, where appropriate.
3. When service user information is required for clinical audit it must be presented in anonymous form to protect confidentiality. Anonymous form means that any means of identifying the service user is removed.
4. The confidentiality of other service users in a project/home must be respected. Therefore, confidential or identifiable information must not be entered into any other service users' records. The use of initials may be used.
5. Confidentiality may be breached if the service user is believed to be at risk to themselves or others or if the organisation is subpoenaed to provide evidence in a court of law.
6. The rights to confidentiality can be waived if the information regarding a service user is required either by National Health Services (NHS) or by any organisation outside the NHS, for example social services, probation officers etc., then the following guidance known as The Caldicott Principles should apply.

3.11   The Caldicott Principles

The Caldicott Principles set out a number of general principles that health and social care organisations should use when reviewing its use of client information.

1. Formal justification of purpose
   Every proposed use or transfer of personally identifiable information within or from an organization should be clearly defined and scrutinized, with continuing uses regularly reviewed by the appropriate guardian.
2. Information transferred
   Information should be transferred only when absolutely necessary. Personally identifiable information items should not be used unless there is no alternative
3. Only the minimum required
   Where the use of personally identifiable information is considered to be essential, each individual item of information should be justified with the aim of reducing identifiability.
4. Need to know access controls

Only those individuals who need access to personally identifiable information should have access to it and they should only have access to the information items that they need to see

5. All understand their responsibilities

   Action should be taken to ensure that those handling personally identifiable information are aware of their responsibilities and obligations to respect patient/service user confidentiality.

6. Comply with and understand the law

   > Every use of personally identifiable information must be lawful. Someone in each organisation should be responsible for ensuring that the organisation complies with legal requirements. Known as the Caldicott guardian (a Caldicott guardian is a senior person responsible for protecting the confidentiality of patient and service-user information and enabling appropriate information-sharing).
   >
   > Caldicott Committee: *Report on the Review of Patient-identifiable Information*, December 1997

3.11.1 Exceptions to the Caldicott Principles

The list of statutory legislation that provides an exception for confidentiality in health information includes:

- Public Health (Control of Diseases) Act 1984 – provides a duty to report the details of a person suffering from a notifiable disease or food poisoning;
- National Health Service Act 1977 – provides duty on a child's father or mother or guardian to notify birth or stillbirth to authority;
- Abortions Regulations 1991 – duty to medical practitioners to notify abortions carried out and any further information needed;
- Prevention of Terrorism Act 1989 – provides power to require the production of information from any person. It is an offence to withhold any such information.

3.12 When access to information should be denied

If a service user requests access to any data held on them, the request must be made in writing to the home/project manager of the care setting they live in and no reason need be given. The applicant must be given a copy of the information and if appropriate an explanation.

In exceptional circumstances information may be withheld:

1. where permitting access to the data would be likely to cause serious harm to the physical condition of the data subject or any other person (which may include a health care professional);
2. where information has been provided by someone else on a confidential basis, and disclosing the data would reveal information which relates to and identifies another person, unless that person has given, signed written consent to release this information;

3. if the request is made by another on behalf of the subject such as parent for a child, access can be refused if the subject has either provided the information in the expectation that it would not be disclosed;
4. if the information is subject to legal privilege or statutory order;
5. the decision to refuse access to information must be by all professionals involved in the service user's care; the reasons for this decision must be clearly documented in the service user's notes.

3.13   Storage and transportation of information

1. Information must be stored in an area that ensures that neither other service users, members of the public or unauthorised members of staff can gain access to them.
2. Where information is stored in areas that do not have 24-hour staff presence, they must be stored in an area that can be securely locked when the premises are unstaffed.
3. If information needs to be transported from one care setting area to another, it is the responsibility of the staff member to ensure that at no point could the information be accessed by unauthorised individuals.
4. It is the staff members' responsibility to ensure that any information is stored safely and securely whilst in transit.

3.14   Computer-held information

1. All computer information held or transmitted are subject to the same controls as manually held information under the Data Protection Act (1998).
2. If information is to be transmitted by fax/email: the member of staff choosing this method of communication is responsible for ensuring that all information transmitted remains confidential.
3. All computer-held information must be password protected and only accessible by authorised users.

3.15   Request for information by and from other agencies

Organisations can disclose personal data to third parties where a service user has given their written consent. Before disclosing the information, staff (Caldicott guardian) should ascertain:

- that the request is actually from the organisation making the request;
- that the request is reasonable, proportionate and relevant (Caldicott principle);
- that the identity of the person making the request is entitled to the data;
- that each time a request is made for personal information for a service user, a record must be kept of the name of the person and the agency who requested the information and the reason for the request and whether the information was given.

All stages of the request must be documented.

3.16   Learning outcomes

- To explain confidentiality in the workplace
- To put the knowledge of confidentiality to everyday work practice
- To ensure that the confidentiality of service users is adhered to according to the organisation's policies
- To relate to any organisation's policies on confidentiality to legislation and law

3.17   Framework for reflective practice

- ➢ *Knowledge*:   What have you learnt from reading this chapter?
- ➢ *Skills:*   What do you know, or can do differently now, that you did not/could not do before reading this chapter?
- ➢ *Practices:*   How can you perform a task now better than before?

3.18   References

Biestek, F.P. (1961) *The Casework Relationship*. London: Allen & Unwin.

British Medical Association (1999) *Confidentiality and Disclosure of Health Information*. London: BMA.

Department for Constitutional Affairs (2007) *Mental Capacity Act 2005: Code of Practice*. London: Department for Constitutional Affairs.

Department of Health (1997) *The Caldicott Committee – Report on The Review of Patient- Identifiable Information*. London: DoH.

Department of Health (2003) *Confidentiality: NHS Code of Practice*. London: DoH.

General Medical Council (2000) *Confidentiality: Protecting and Providing Information*. London: GMC.

General Social Care Council (2002) *Code of Practice for Social Care Workers and Code of Practice for Employers of Social Care Workers*. London: GSCC.

Health Professions Council (2003) *Standards of Conduct, Performance and Ethics*. London: HPC.

HMSO (1998) *Children's Act 1989*. London: HMSO.

HMSO (1998) *Data Protection Act 1998*. London: HMSO.

HMSO (1998) *Human Rights Act 1998*. London: HMSO.

HMSO (2001) *Health and Social Care Act 2001*. London: HMSO.

HMSO (2005) *Mental Capacity Act 2005*. London: HMSO.

National Health Service (2010) *Consent and Disclosure Guidelines*. (www.elf.nelft.nhs.uk)

Thomson, N. (2000) *Understanding Social Work*. Basingstoke: Macmillan Press.

Thompson, N. and Thompson, S. (2008) *The Social Work Companion*. London: Palgrave Macmillan.

3.19   Induction workbook

1. Confidentiality is important because;

   _____

   _____

2. Give three examples when confidential information may need to be shared explaining why.

   _____

   _____

3. Identify six ways of maintaining confidentiality in the workplace on a daily basis.

    _____

    _____

4. How can confidentiality be breached at your place of work?

    _____

    _____

5. What is confidentiality?

    _____

    _____

6. In what circumstances might you have to break confidentiality?

    _____

    _____

7. What do the Caldicott Principles state in relation to confidentiality?

    _____

    _____

8. Research how all types of information must be stored to maintain confidentiality

    _____

    _____

9. Identify the impact a breach of confidentiality may have on an organisation or an individual

    _____

    _____

4   Professional Boundaries

AIMS

➢ To understand the concept of boundaries in health and social care and why we have them

➢ To understand what professional boundaries are and their importance

➢ To recognise ways in which professional boundaries may be breached, and what may be done if they are breached

➢ To use boundaries in our professional relationships

➢ To identify the difference between a professional relationship and a non-professional relationship

4.1   Introduction

Boundaries are found in all areas of our lives – socially, economically, politically, physically, emotionally and even spiritually. They are important because they define the limits and responsibilities of the people with whom we interact, which mark our personal boundaries. Similarly, we have boundaries in employment and whilst the basic boundaries in employment are similar in many sectors, the application, understanding and maintenance of boundaries in the field of health and social care are more complex because of the relationship that social care workers hold with their service users, the amount of time they spend with the service users, and the nature of the subjects they deal with; hence the establishment of professional guidelines which define professional boundaries that add structure to the relationship between service user and social care worker.

These boundaries guide a social care worker on how to engender empathy and warmth, while retaining a clear professional boundary. It is clear that a lack of clarity at the outset has the potential to create real problems and unless social care workers understand why these boundaries are there, they could find themselves involved in a difficult situation and not know how to cope, giving the service user the wrong idea, which could cause pain and distress to the service user, themselves and the team. The social care worker may enter into a relationship of 'caring about' rather than 'caring for' the service user.

This chapter provides a structured induction literature in professional boundaries, for those employed through the recruitment agencies with no formal training to work in health and social care and those already working in the sector who have not received any formal training on professional boundaries. However, given the lack of detailed training in the sector on boundaries, it is suitable for people at all stages of their career as a refresher or to top up on their existing knowledge, or those in transition from other sectors like factories into health and social care. Boundaries are an area on which it is always worth reflecting in order to improve safe practice and improve on the quality of care.

4.2   What is a professional boundary in healthcare?

A boundary in healthcare is defined as the limits of behaviour, which allow staff to have professional relationships with service users receiving care and/or treatment from them. These boundaries are based upon trust, respect and the appropriate use of power. (NE London, NHS Foundation Trust)

4.3   Types of staff–service user relationship

4.3.1   Direct relationships

This is where a caregiver, support worker or healthcare assistant (staff), either individually or as part of a team, is providing a service directly to a service user as part of their normal duties, e.g. personal care, key working, link work, housing management services or similar roles. Managers of staff in these situations should also be deemed to be in a direct relationship with service users.

4.3.2   Indirect relationships

This is where a staff member comes into contact with the service user on some basis which is not connected to the direct provision of support or service delivery. Indirect contact will include:

- working with a service user in day services or similar representatives like garden centres;
- managing volunteer; or
- work placement where the service user is receiving primary services elsewhere. e.g. drug rehabilitation.

4.3.3   Professional relationships

A professional relationship may be defined as a relationship which involves planned and goal-orientated interactions between the staff and the service user, with the aim of providing help to the service user. A professional relationship that is appropriate focuses exclusively upon the needs of the service user.

4.3.4   Professional working relationships

In indirect relationships, following a risk assessment by a team leader or line manager, there may be need to share confidential information with service users on work or volunteer placement, provided it will facilitate the performance of their normal duties. The service user, however, must be made aware of their duty of confidentiality not to disclose any data they may come across with third parties without proper consent of the management of the work placement.

In order to maintain professional working relationships, staff should:

- never disclose inappropriate personal information about themselves such as history of previous addictions, offences or financial status, their home address, personal mobile/home telephone numbers, personal email addresses, details about their family or life outside of work;
- never ask service users for personal information that is unrelated to their support needs;

- never disclose personal information about other service users or third parties, in line with the organisation's confidentiality and privacy policy;
- always respect service users' rights to dignity, empower them to be able to make choices and to be treated fairly, irrespective of their race, ethnicity, gender, sexual orientation, age, disability, religious belief or lack of it or other characteristics unique to them;
- never take service users to their homes;
- avoid breaching professional boundaries by smoking with the service users as a tool to engaging with them during key working sessions;
- never be complicit in nor engage in illegal activities with service users nor encourage them to do so – for example, smoking cannabis;

Staff who encounter service users out of hours should be pleasant and civil if approached by the service user, but should generally discourage prolonged social contact. Staff should not approach service users in any social setting if the contact is not instigated by the service user, especially where the service user's behaviour indicates that they do not want to be recognised or identified as a user of the service.

4.3.5   Sexual relationships

Staff should be aware that dress code is important in maintaining boundaries. Inappropriate clothing may send messages to others without any verbal encouragement. Employers are responsible for ensuring that an appropriate dress code is observed by their staff. Therefore:

- staff must never knowingly enter into intimate or sexual relationships with service users in whatever capacity except in the situations where an intimate relationship with someone who becomes a service user; however, the employer must be notified immediately; the staff–service user relationship should be on an indirect basis only and the staff member concerned should not be involved in any decision-making or key-working regarding that service user;
- staff should never respond to or engage in flirting with service users, whether innocent or otherwise;
- staff should immediately declare to their employer if they enter into an intimate relationship with a service user or with an individual who they subsequently discover is a service user; this is in order to prevent any potential or inherent conflicts of interest, exploitation of vulnerable people or abuse of trust;
- it is unacceptable for staff to engage in improper behaviour which could lead to a sexual relationship developing, as this would be seen as abuse of trust and exploitation of a vulnerable person – such as those with learning or sensory disabilities or those who have been in an abusive relationship; these people are especially dependent on relationship of trust with staff;
- where staff come into contact with a service user with whom they have had an intimate relationship prior to entering employment with the service provider, this should be declared immediately to the employer; in this case, a direct working relationship with that service user should not be permitted, such as key-working.

4.3.6   Non-professional relationships

A non-professional relationship may be defined as a social relationship which is casual, friendly or romantic. The relationship has equal balance of power and is for the mutual interest and pleasure for both parties involved.

4.4   Types of boundaries

There are four types of boundaries that govern relationships in the health and social care environment: general, financial, verbal and physical boundaries. Boundaries may also include emotional or spiritual boundaries. They can consist of the limits of what we consider safe and appropriate, our unique set of feelings and reactions, individual perceptions, values, goals, concerns, roles we choose to play. However, in a health and social care environment, these boundaries define professional behaviour.

4.4.1   General boundaries

General boundaries create order and define our rolls of interaction with the service users. For example, in direct relationships boundaries are based upon absolute trust and professional integrity. Whereas boundaries in indirect relationships are important, the nature of the relationship needs to be fully considered within the context of a risk assessment when deciding whether a particular boundary can be relaxed, e.g. working with service users in garden centres, day centres or work placements.

However, whether a boundary concerns a direct or indirect relationship in a health and social care setting, dignity in the workplace should be paramount and all conflicts of interests must be declared to the relevant management, e.g. where a staff member knows a service user from another context such as having attended the same school, a risk assessment should be made about managing the conflict, if applicable.

4.4.2   Financial boundaries and gifts

In order to maintain a professional relationship where money or gifts are concerned, staff should:

- never buy items from service users or sell items to them unless this is on behalf of the organisation they are working for;
- never lend money or personal property to service users;
- always write out a dated receipt for any financial transactions with the service user to avoid any impression that a personal, financial or material benefit could be derived from them;
- never accept cash gifts from service users, unless this is a donation to the project/ residential home welfare scheme for which a receipt should be given;
- never encourage service users to include them in their wills or last testaments nor agree to become trustees, beneficiaries or executors in relation to the wills of service users;
- never accept or solicit personal gifts or rewards from service users;
- never make personal gifts or donations to service users; all gifts must only be made on behalf of the organisation.

4.4.3   Verbal boundaries

In order to maintain a professional relationship in a care environment:

- staff must always treat service users fairly, courteously and with respect in accordance with laid down organisations' communication policy, values, the equality and diversity policy;
- staff should never use language which is discriminatory, demeaning, sexually suggestive or insulting or which could be perceived as such;
- staff should be seen as approachable, open to fair challenge and criticism, and available to engage in meaningful dialogue;
- staff should not be seen as intimidating or inaccessible people; service users must not be discouraged from accessing support within agreed boundaries or from making complaints;
- staff should be careful not to use overly familiar language, endearments or nicknames with service users nor should they encourage service users to address them or other colleagues using such language; this is in order to avoid the risk of eroding professional relationships;
- staff should never give medical advice to service users but always refer medical problems to qualified health professionals.

4.4.4   Physical boundaries

> Physical boundaries refer to the area around a person (personal space), which is generally 2.5 to 3 feet. (Crisis Prevention Institute, 2001)

In normal settings, offering someone physical support through touch/contact, is often seen as a humane or sympathetic way of dealing with someone's joy or distress. However, touch/contact in the work of a social care worker with the service users can be seen as preventing the healing process, so alternative verbal or nonverbal communication modes can be far more effective.

In the health and social care environment, there is always a likelihood of allegations being made against social care worker because of inappropriate or misconstrued physical contact. Some service users may misinterpret physical contact as affection outside the professional relationship, while others may see physical contact as expressions of favouritism, for example where a staff member hugs one service user and not another

This, however, is dependent upon the nature of services the organisation offers and the nature of the service user groups using the services. Where touching does occur it should take place within the specific local work instructions or professional boundaries within the service.

Hence, organisations should require all staff including volunteer workers to:

- avoid any physical contact other than shaking hands, or similar social conventions between strangers or people who do not know each other well; a handshake creates a degree of safety and strengthens boundaries and people's awareness of them;
- avoid invading someone's personal space if this could be misunderstood by the service user or seen as threatening; be aware of personal space, which is the distance of the arm's length of an outstretched hand;

- never administer first aid without having attended a recognised training course;
- relate Breakaway techniques (training) (see Section 11.15.10, p. 222) to professional boundaries; physical contact should only be used for defensive purposes only – to break free of a problematic situation; retaliation, physical punishment and physical restraint are unacceptable; unreasonable physical restraint by a member of staff who may be stronger than a service user and untrained may lead to injury.

Physical contact should only be used if it is set as part of intervention plan, and protocols should be set as part of a care plan for service users with challenging behaviour by the multidisciplinary team and should only be used by trained members of staff.

Where service users initiate contact – for example, by throwing their arms around a staff member – staff must slowly and politely break free. Whilst doing so, it is recommended that eye contact and supportive conversation be maintained. The service user's hands should be held in front until it is appropriate to let go completely.

4.5   What is a professional boundary?

A professional boundary may be defined as a set of instructions, principles, expectations and rules which set the ethical standards in the health and social care environment. They set limits of the professional behaviour that allow for a safe, effective and appropriate therapeutic interaction between the professionals and the service users based upon trust, respect and the appropriate use of power.

It is staff's responsibility to maintain their professional and personal boundaries as well as to assist colleagues and service users in maintaining theirs.

> The staff member knows what constitutes appropriate professional practice, whereas the Service User or Carer is in an unfamiliar situation and may not know what is appropriate.
> (CHRE – Council for Healthcare Regulatory Excellence, 2008)

4.6   Why do we have professional boundaries?

In the health and social care environment, selection and maintenance of appropriate boundaries in a staff–service user relationship facilitate safe and therapeutic practice. Setting and maintaining boundaries should also be seen as part of the standard expectations of staff, agencies and regulators as well as upholding the service provider's (organisation) values statement.

Professional boundaries are there to:

- protect the space between the professional's power and the service user's vulnerability; it is important that staff be aware of the power imbalance that exists in the professional relationship between staff and the service user; this power imbalance is generated by the service user's need for care, assistance and support and places them in a position of vulnerability if trust is not respected;
- enable staff to better undertake their role by striking the right balance between compassion and professionalism;
- help staff maintain an effective professional relationship with the service user in such a way that it is therapeutic for the service user;

- help staff to deliver fair service to service users without accusations of favouritism, as boundaries clarify the role of the worker, how they are going to work with the service user and what the service user should expect them to achieve;
- help to ensure maximum benefits of care to the service users and focus exclusively upon the needs of the service user;
- help professionals manage themselves and their emotions so they can show empathy and how to engender empathy and warmth, while retaining a clear professional boundary;
- protect staff/volunteers from undue pressure or allegations from service users;
- enable staff to provide consistency across all organisations activities.

4.7   How to use boundaries in our professional relationships

A model which can be used to illustrate the range of professional behaviour is the Continuum of Professional Behaviour (National Council of State Boards of Nursing, 1996), where the majority of interactions between a nurse and a person in their care should occur for effectiveness and the safety of that person. This model identifies three zones:

- zone of under-involvement
- zone of over-involvement
- zone of helpfulness

4.7.1   Zone of under-involvement

This refers to those activities and behaviours that lead to and include neglect and assault. Staff practising in this zone of under-involvement may be too cold, distant, or formal and not caring enough to be helpful to the service user.

4.7.2   Zone of over-involvement

This zone refers to 'caring about' rather than 'caring for' the client. This may lead to a situation where the relationship between the staff and the client takes priority over the client's care needs. Staff practising in this zone of over-involvement may be overly-involved, too 'touchy-feely' or intrusive.

4.7.3   Zone of helpfulness

This zone refers to the activities and behaviour that result in safe and effective staff/service user care. In order to maintain practice within the zone of helpfulness, staff need to be aware of the professional boundaries in relation to staff–client relationship, and act in accordance with these at all times. See Figure 4.1.

4.8   Ways in which professional boundaries may be breached

A boundary may be breached by any behaviour or interaction which physically, emotionally or economically harms the staff or service user.

Staff may breach boundaries in one of two ways.

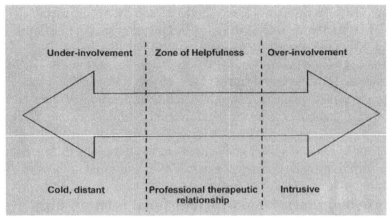

Figure 4.1 Model illustrating the continuum of professional behaviour.

4.8.1   Boundary crossing

This is where staff make a conscious decision to deviate from the established boundaries of the usual framework of practice, but their action does not exploit or harm the patient. Rather, it may enhance the therapeutic relationship if the boundary is crossed to meet a therapeutic need – for example, disclosing personal information to the service user to empathise with them, or providing reassurance or building rapport.

> However, when it comes to self-disclosure, you need to ask yourself? How will this self-disclosure benefit in meeting the client's health care needs? Is the self-disclosure consistent with the care plan? (National Council of State Boards of Nursing [NCSBN], 2011)

4.8.2   Boundary violation

> A boundary violation is typically characterized by a reversal of roles, secrecy, the creation of a double bind for the client and the indulgence of personal privilege by the professional (College & Association of Registered Nurses of Alberta (CARNA), 2005, p. 5).

Boundary violation means the misuse of power or the betrayal of trust, respect or intimacy between staff and service user. Violations of boundary can include inappropriate personal questioning, inappropriate touch/contact, attempting to control how the service user thinks, believes, or feels. This can cause physical, emotional and/or economical harm to the service user. An example of boundary violation is attempting to combine a non-professional (social) and professional (therapeutic) relationship with the service user.

4.9   How to maintain professional boundaries

4.9.1   How to reflect on your behaviour

It is clear that a lack of clarity and training in professional boundaries for the role of social care workers has the potential to create real problems. Unless social care workers understand why these boundaries are there, they could find themselves involved in a difficult situation and not know how to cope, giving service users the wrong ideas, which could cause pain and distress to themselves and the team and result in self-injurious behaviour for the service user.

4.9.2 Questions to ask yourself

To be successful at establishing and maintaining therapeutic relationships, health and social care workers must ask themselves questions to help them reflect on their behaviour within the staff-service user relationship:

- Is my behaviour in the service user's best interest?
- Whose needs are being served (mine or the service users')?
- What impact will my behaviour have on the service I am delivering?
- How would my behaviour be viewed by the service user's family or other colleagues?
- Am I comfortable telling colleagues about my behaviour?
- Am I comfortable documenting my behaviour in the service user's daily diary?
- Am I treating this service user differently (e.g. extent of personal disclosure)?
- Does this service user mean something 'special' to me?
- Am I taking advantage of the service user?
- Does my behaviour breach any of the organisation's care policies or standards?

4.10 The consequences of breaching professional boundaries

It is essential that staff conduct themselves in accordance with the professional boundaries relating to staff–service user relationships and be aware of the serious consequences of the extreme violations of professional boundaries. This will help avoid:

- potential or actual harm to staff and/service users through violence against staff or physical restraints by untrained staff;
- reduced level of care for the service user, for example, not giving medication on time or being given too much medication by untrained carers;
- breakdown in therapeutic relationship;
- staff abusing service users' vulnerability – through physical abuse or emotional neglect by ignoring or excluding them from conversation;
- creating emotional dependence for service users.

4.11 Guidelines to avoid breaching professional boundaries

4.11.1 Individual responsibilities

Staff should:
- read, understand and follow professional code of conduct and code of ethics;
- adhere to organisation's policies and procedures on professional boundaries;
- define limits of confidentiality with the service user;
- avoid inappropriate self-disclosure to service users;
- employ regular self-assessment on boundary issues;

- share information with their colleagues;
- resist flattery and flirtation;
- understand the difficulties of the service users they work with and the implications for them;
- avoid dual (therapeutic and social) relationships with the service user as far as possible;
- adhere to the plans of care;
- communicate the expectations for and limits of confidentiality;
- be sensitive to the context in which the care is provided;
- implement reflective practice.

4.11.2 Team responsibilities

Staff should:

- maintain team contact and offer support to avoid other team members becoming isolated and vulnerable at work;
- help colleagues – since boundary violations are usually unintended, staff are often not aware they have crossed a boundary;
- request mandatory formal debrief after a serious incident involving a breach in professional boundaries;
- ensure discussions of boundary related issues are a regular topic in staff meetings, e.g. the reason the service users try to gain intimacy with staff;
- request and use regular staff supervision to discuss boundary-related issues;
- acquire training and information on boundary issues from their organisation or other sources like books, websites and journals.

4.12 Self-assessment questionnaire

- ❑ Have you had difficulties setting and adhering to professional boundaries in your staff-service user relationship?
- ❑ Have you felt that another member of staff was too critical of 'your' service user?
- ❑ Have you felt you are the only one who understands a particular service user, and/or been jealous of other staff's relationship with a service user?
- ❑ Have you found yourself relating to a service user as you would a family member?
- ❑ Have you received feedback from anyone that you are overly involved with a service user?
- ❑ Have you kept secrets or felt that there were things about a service user that you did not want to share with other staff?
- ❑ Have you ever tried punishing a service user (e.g. by withdrawing something they were entitled to)?
- ❑ Have you ever deliberately hurt a service user during physical restraint?
- ❑ Have you ever shouted in anger at a service user?
- ❑ Have you ever found it difficult to handle a service user's request for assistance, verbal abuse or sexual language because of issues from your own experiences?

❑ Do you feel uncomfortable in approaching your colleagues or team leader/manager to discuss your feelings about a service user?

4.13 Warning signs that professional boundaries have been or have the potential to be breached

- Having unrealistic expectations of your relationship with the service user (for example to 'rescue' them or 'heal them with love').
- You are not comfortable sharing your actions with others or recording them.
- Spending time with a service user out of work hours.
- Frequently thinking about a service user when you are away from work.
- There is more physical touching than is appropriate or sexual content in interaction with a service user.
- Favouring one service user at the expense of another service user.
- Changing which service user you are assigned to work with in a large setting.
- Selective reporting of service user's behaviour, i.e. positive or negative service user's behaviour.
- Acting and/or feeling possessive about a particular service user.
- Giving special attention/treatment to a service user which differs from that given to other service users.
- Treating service users as personal friends.
- Trying to satisfy your personal needs via the service user.
- Keeping secrets with the service user.
- Sharing personal information or work concerns with service users.

4.14 Indicators of boundary breaches

Indicators of boundary breaches inform staff how to recognise actual or potential practice outside of the zone of safe practice, i.e. zone of helpfulness.

4.14.1 Therapeutic relationships

Staff need to recognise their own values and service users' values and the potential for value conflict, and act in a way that does not diminish care of the service user.

Indicators of boundary breaches that may be evident in this category include:

1. *Presence of:*
   - judgmental attitudes – being critical of the service user;
   - co-dependence relationships;
   - rudeness/patronising behaviour;
   - favouritism/minimal care/neglect;
   - roughness/bullying/assault;
   - possessive/secretive behaviour.

2.   *Absence/lack of:*
- sensitivity;
- individualised assessment of care;
- being there for the service user;
- awareness of service users' rights;
- concern/understanding/listening;
- effective communication.

4.14.2 Access to/disclosure of information

A degree of self-disclosure may be appropriate for the development of trust and building rapport in the staff–service user relationship. However, deciding on the appropriate balance for the self-disclosure or non-disclosure must be based on the service user's needs.

The use of self-disclosure as a debriefing strategy for staff's own unresolved issues is always inappropriate and potentially harmful to the service user. Therefore, the provision of adequate information (for example, about aspect of care) can empower service users and impact positively on their care experience.

Indicators of boundary breaches that may be present in this category may include:

- staff may closely identify with a service user's experience;
- dual relationships may exist with the service user or significant others in service user's life;
- staff may be experiencing difficulties with unresolved issues in their personal life;
- early self-disclosure may inhibit the formation of a staff–service user professional relationship.

4.14.3 Dual relationships

Dual relationships occur when health and social care workers relate to service users in more than one relationship, whether professional, social, or business. Dual relationships occur simultaneously or consecutively.

The creation of platonic, non-sexual or sexual relationships during a therapeutic relationship increases service users' vulnerability. Therefore, it is of paramount importance to ensure that the staff–service user relationship is always conducted with the sole intent of benefiting the service user.

Indicators of boundary breach that may be present in this category include:

- self-disclosure or inappropriate behaviour;
- the service user is aware of the change in the nature of the relationship that is no longer professional;
- potential harm to the service user and/or staff with the ongoing professional interaction;
- issues relating to confidentiality may be violated.

4.14.4 Giving and receiving gifts

Staff should be aware that the giving and receiving of gifts within the staff-service user relationship has the potential to compromise the professional relationship.

The following factors can be used to assess the appropriateness of the gift transaction:

- Timing – has the gift been given before, during, or after provision of care?
- Consequences – what are the implications e.g. family response, discomfort accepting or refusing the gift?
- Intent – was the gift coerced from the service user? Is there an expectation of different care?
- Personal gain – what is the relative value to the giver and the recipient?
- Cultural/religious factors need to be considered when assessing how to deal with acceptance or refusal of a gift.

4.15 Prevention of sexual misconduct

Sexual misconduct encompasses a range of behaviours used to obtain sexual gratification against another's will or at the expense of another. Sexual misconduct includes sexual harassment, sexual assault, and any conduct of a sexual nature that is without consent, or has the effect of threatening or intimidating the person against whom such conduct is directed. State laws vary on defining acts which constitute sexual misconduct (legal definition).

There are usually guidelines, training and clear policies to help staff/volunteers workers prevent sexual misconduct within the staff–service user relationship in a care environment.

4.15.1 Do's

- ✓ Respect cultural differences and be aware of the sensitivities of individual service users.
- ✓ Learn to detect and appropriately deflect service users' inappropriate sexual behaviour, and control the support environment.
- ✓ Offer appropriate supportive contact when warranted.
- ✓ Maintain accurate records that reflect any intimate questions of a sexual nature, and document all comments or concerns made by the service user relating to alleged sexual abuse.

4.15.2 Don'ts

- ✖ Do not use gesture, tone of voice, expressions, or any other behaviour which a service user may interpret as seductive, sexually demeaning or sexually abusive.
- ✖ Do not make inappropriate sexualised comments about or to a service user.
- ✖ Do not ask details about the service user's sexual history or sexual likes and dislikes unless directly related to the purposes of the consultation.
- ✖ Do not criticise a service user's sexual preferences.
- ✖ Do not engage in inappropriate sexual behaviour with a service user, including requesting a date, hugging, touching, kissing and sexual intercourse.
- ✖ Do not talk about your own sexual preferences, fantasies, problems or activities or performances with service users.

4.16 Summary

- A professional boundary may be defined as a set of instructions, principles, expectations and rules which set the ethical standards in the health and social care environment.
- A boundary may be breached by any behaviour or interaction which physically, emotionally or economically harms the staff or service user.
- It is staff's responsibility to maintain professional boundaries within the therapeutic relationship at all times. The staff member knows what constitutes appropriate professional practice, whereas the service user or carer is in an unfamiliar situation and may not know what is appropriate (CHRE, 2008).
- A professional therapeutic relationship may be defined as a relationship which involves planned and goal-oriented interactions between staff and service user, with the aim of providing help to the service user.
- The Zone of Helpfulness refers to activities and behaviour that result in safe and effective staff/client care. In order to maintain practice within the Zone of Helpfulness, staff need to be aware of professional boundaries in relation to staff–client relationships, and act in accordance with these at all times.

4.17 Learning outcomes

- To maintain the appropriate boundaries of staff relationships, and to help service users understand when their requests are beyond the limits of the professional relationship.
- To develop and follow a comprehensive care plan with the service users on professional boundaries.
- To ensure that any approach or activity that could be perceived as a boundary violation is included in the care plan developed by the multidisciplinary care team.
- To recognise that there may be an increased need for vigilance in maintaining professionalism and boundaries in certain practice settings, e.g. during massage sessions.
- To reduce professional isolation by maintaining regular contact with colleagues, reflecting on professional relationships with peers and participating in formal supervision.

4.18 Framework for reflective practice

- ➢ *Knowledge:*   What have you learnt from reading this chapter?
- ➢ *Skills:*   What do you know, or can do differently now, that you did not/could not do before reading this chapter?
- ➢ *Practices:*   How can you perform a task now better than before?

4.19 References

Bateman, N. (2000) *Advocacy Skills for Health and Social Care Professionals*. London: Jessica Kingsley.

Cooper, F. (2012) *Professional Boundaries in Social Work and Social Care: A Practical Guide to Understanding, Maintaining and Managing Your Professional Boundaries*. London: Jessica Kingsley.

Connor, A., MacLennan, E. and Price, S. (2009) *HNC in Social Care Student Book*. London: Heinemann.

Council for Healthcare Regulatory Excellence (2008) *Clear Sexual Boundaries between Healthcare Professionals and Patients: Responsibilities of Healthcare Professionals.* London: CHRE,

Department of Health (2002) *Code of Conduct for Managers Guidelines.* London: DoH.

Division of Clinical Psychology of the British Psychology Society (1999) *Professional Practice Guidelines.* London: British Psychology Society.

General Social Care Council (2002) *Codes of Practice for Social Care Workers and Employers.* London: GSCC. Available at http://www.skilsforcare.org.uk/codes/

General Social Care Council (2004) *Code of Practice.* London: GSCC.

General Social Care Council (2008*) Raising Standards: Social Work Conduct in England.* London: GSCC. Available at: http://www.skillsforcare.org.uk

General Social Care Council (2009) *Raising Standards: Social Work Conduct in England 2003–2008.* London: GSCC.

Halter, M., Brown, H. and Stone, J. (2007) *Sexual Boundary Violations by Health Professional – An Overview of the Published Empirical Literature.* Council for Healthcare Regulatory Excellence

Hardy, B., Hudson, B. and Waddington, E. (2000) *What Makes a Good Partnership? A Partnership Assessment Tool.* Leeds: Nuffield Institute for Health.

Haug, I.E. (1999) Boundaries and the use and misuse of power and authority: ethical complexities for clergy psychotherapists, *Journal of Counselling and Development* 77: 411–17.

Kabel, J.D. and Giebelhausen, P.N. (1994) Dual relationships and professional boundaries, *Social Work* **39**(2): 213–20.

National Council of State Boards of Nursing (1996) *Continuum of Professional Behaviour.* London: NCSBN.

Nursing and Midwifery Council (2002) *Code of Professional Conduct.* London: NMC.

Nursing and Midwifery Council (2002) *Practitioner and Client Relationships and the Prevention of Abuse.* London: NMC.

Nursing and Midwifery Council (2008) *The Code.* London: NMC.

Thompson, N. and Thompson, S. (2008) *The Social Work Companion.* London: Palgrave Macmillan.

Whitfield, C.L. (1993) *Boundaries and Relationships: Knowing, Protecting, and Enjoying the Self.* Deerfield Beach, FL: Health Communications, Inc.

4.20   Induction workbook

1. Describe the limitations of a professional relationship with a service user and importance of professional boundaries.

2. How can professional boundaries be breached?

    _____

    _____

3. In what ways is staff relationship different from the relationship with the service user?

    _____

    _____

4. What are the main indicators that professional boundaries have been breached?

    _____

    _____

5. What is self-disclosure? What effect can it have on the self-user?

    _____

    _____

6. Define professional boundary and state how it differs from professional relationship.

    _____

    _____

7. List at least six indicators that indicate that professional boundaries have been or have the potential to be breached.

    _____

    _____

8. What do you understand by The Public Interest Disclosure Act 1998? And what issues are raised under the Confidential Reporting Policy?

    _____

    _____

9. Outline the various types of boundaries and how they can be breached and explain ways in which this can be prevented

    _____

    _____

10. Describe the environment under which professional boundaries can be breached and how it can be prevented.

    _____

    _____

PART II

THE ORGANISATION AND YOUR ROLE

5 Social Care Worker's Role in the Organisation

AIMS

➢ To understand your job role and responsibilities, including an awareness of the role of others and how to work in partnership with them

➢ To understand the need to work in line with policies and procedures

5.1 Characteristics of a good social care worker

The main purpose of a social care worker is to provide high-quality care services to service users and to maintain their respect and dignity at all times. A good social care worker requires:

- good communication skills;
- good interpersonal skills;
- resourcefulness – being able to identify and take measures to reduce anxiety;
- discretion;
- trustworthiness/integrity;
- motivation to learn and improve professional skills;
- commitment;
- good judgment skills;
- ability to advocate on behalf of someone else (service users);
- a good team player.

5.2 Job description

A job description outlines the role, in terms of both the day-to-day tasks and responsibilities and includes:

- the position of the job within the organisation as a whole;
- the geographical location and setting of the job;
- the day-to-day tasks and duties which make up the bulk of the job;
- any occasional duties, for example travel or covering for others;
- any special working conditions, for example shift work, unusual hours, travel;
- other benefits, for example holiday entitlement, pension schemes, childcare facilities, flexible working hours, career breaks, accommodation of religious breaks, adaptable working uniform, prayer space and time.

5.3 Job summary

A job summary is a brief, general statement of the more important functions and responsibilities of a job (BusinessDictionary.com)

Job summary of a support worker, healthcare assistant, project worker or caregiver:

1. To support the service users including adults and young people with learning difficulties, housing needs, complex needs (such as those involved in substance misuse), mental health issues and asylum seekers, in all areas of their lives.
2. To help promote a stimulating, caring and culturally appropriate environment for the service users.
3. To provide practical and emotional support to enable the service users under the guidance of the management team led a fulfilling life.
4. To work closely with the service users, their families and representative to implement all care plans agreed upon.
5. To work within, and promote, the policies and procedures of service providers.

5.4 Main duties and general responsibilities

To participate in a full range of caring duties including:

- helping service users with leisure interests and skill development inside and outside their residential settings;
- establishing a rapport with the service user and you as a staff member;
- providing personal care to service users, enabling them to look clean and attractive;
- implementing personal care plans set out for the service users;
- helping service users to keep their possessions and living areas clean, tidy and safe;
- domestic duties including washing, cleaning, cooking etc.;
- communicating with other staff about service users' needs and activities;
- recording service user's needs/activities/behaviour in their daily diaries according to record- keeping policy;
- to help ensure that each service user's health needs have been met including:

  o liaising with medical services (e.g. GP, dentist, chiropodist);
  o ensuring the implementation of appropriate medication procedures.

5.5 Key work

5.5.1 What is key work?

Key work is the process through which a service user, and the staff allocated to work as their key worker, work together to identify their needs, and to agree and achieve their goals. At each key work session the service user and key worker should measure the progress and look at areas in which the service user may still need help.

5.5.2 Duties of a key worker

- Being responsible for anticipating service users' needs and communicating these needs to other staff and professionals involved with the service user.
- Being involved in writing review reports and other reports necessary for that service user.

- Being involved in setting up and implementing personal care plans for that service user.
- Being involved in review meetings concerning that service user.
- Listening to service users, including their feelings about any difficulties they may be having.

Key workers help service users express their needs and have them met by:

- establishing good relationships with service user's families and advocates;
- coordinating reviews at least once a year for each service user;
- ensuring up-to-date records are kept for the service user and other documentation, i.e. incident forms, shift planner, activities timetables, organising holidays etc.
- liaison and administration to work closely and in a professional manner with other professionals, both within and outside of the home or project, e.g. social workers and advocates;
- to use communications systems effectively, e.g. diary, communication book and verbally to colleagues;
- implementation of individual program, plans and their ongoing development;
- to work with others to suggest updates to support plans and risk assessments and reporting back to the rest of the team about changes to support plans;
- to review and reconcile bank statements at the end of each month, ensuring an up-to-date financial risk assessment is in place and highlighting issues to the service manager.

5.5.3 Other duties

- To work in a way consistent with the principles of 'normalisation' and 'Equal Opportunities', i.e. to give each service user practical skills and social status that are valued within their communities.
- To have anti-racist and anti-sexist work practices, which help them value anti-discriminatory attitudes and behaviours.
- To act in accordance with all policies and procedures, e.g. health and safety, fire drills.

5.6 The role of project workers in supported housing/shelter projects

The purpose of support services is to help service users to prepare to live independently. The project worker's duties to the service users will include:

- finding the service user education or training with relevant bodies;
- getting a job/work placement/apprenticeships;
- claiming and processing benefits;
- managing finances through budgeting;
- staying healthy and registering with the general practitioner/dentists;
- paying rent and managing tenancy;
- completing forms and keeping appointments;
- moving on to a more permanent place to live;
- referral to agencies dealing with drugs/substances abuse.

5.7   Learning outcomes

- To be able to apply the knowledge-specific needs of your organisation.
- To get started straight away and apply the learning to your work.
- To help you implement the knowledge in the context of the organisation.
- To increase effectiveness, continuous development and lasting change for you and the organisation.

5.8   Framework for reflective practice

➢ *Knowledge:*   What have you learnt from reading this chapter?
➢ *Skills:*   What do you know, or can do differently now, that you did not/could not do before reading this chapter?
➢ *Practices:*   How can you perform a task now better than before?

5.9   Reference

Bateman, N. (2000) *Advocacy Skills for Health and Social Care Professionals*. London, Jessica Kingsley.

5.10   Induction workbook

1. What responsibilities, do you have to service users as a support worker?
   _____
   _____

2. Briefly outline your main responsibilities in a care setting.
   _____
   _____

3. Explain what the aims of the services are.
   _____
   _____

4. Who are the people you will be directly working with?
   _____
   _____

5. Do service users have any responsibilities? Can you name any two?
   _____
   _____

6. Why is it important to involve family and carers in the day-to-day life of service users?

    _____

    _____

7. Why is it important to have a positive approach while working with the service user group, and the individual within the group?

    _____

    _____

8. As a social care worker, how can you demonstrate that you have a positive approach to the lives and experience of service users with whom you will be, or are, working?

    _____

    _____

9. What is key work? And what are the duties of a key worker in relation to the service user in a care setting?

    _____

    _____

10. Identify and explain the duties of project workers in supported housing/shelter to the service users.

    _____

    _____

11. What are the limitations faced by the key worker in any care environment in supporting service users?

    _____

    _____

6   Application of Policies and Procedures

AIMS

➤ To be able to understand and relate to policies and procedure in the workplace

➤ To understand and apply the policies and procedures that are important to your role

➤ To be able to put the knowledge of policies and procedures to everyday work practice

➤ To understand the importance of adhering to the policies and procedures laid down by organisations

➤ To be able to relate to any organisation's policies and procedures to legislation and law

6.1   Introduction

• This chapter gives a general introduction to the care setting and some policies and procedures within which you will be working in the care environment.

6.2   Role of Commission for Social Care Inspection (CSCI)

The Commission for Social Care Inspection (CSCI) is responsible for registering and inspecting social care in England, which includes residential homes for people living with learning disabilities. Part of the CSCI's role is to:

• promote improvement in social care;
• inspect all social care establishments;
• publish annual reports on the performance of social care.

The CSCI inspects residential settings against National Minimum Standards (NMS). These set the regulations which outline how the care setting should be organised, staffed, and run. The CSCI ensures that social care workers, like you are working to agreed standards of care. There are, therefore, guidelines in the form of Code of Practice that you need to be working within. Each of these is a fundamental value which should underpin the way you work in care.

6.3   National Service Frameworks

The government has also produced National Service Frameworks which set out standards and service models to which health and social care services have to adhere and against which they are measured. The intention of these is to improve standards of care and promote closer working relationships between health and social care services.

The induction standards describe the understanding you should have of your role and responsibilities, and how these relate to the organisation's aims and values. It also describes the understanding that you should have to access, understand and use the policies and procedures that are important to your role. It is recognised by organisations that it will not be possible for you to have to understand thoroughly all organisational policies and procedures; however, new staff should at least understand policies and procedures that are important for them to carry out their role properly and safely.

6.4   Policies, procedures and their application

6.4.1   What is a policy?

A policy is a statement that outlines how the organisation will act on a particular issue.

6.4.2   What is a procedure?

A procedure is a step-by-step guide on how to carry out an activity in the workplace.
- Procedures provide guidelines on how to share certain types of information.
- A procedure on grievances or complaints, for example, outlines the step of reporting and resolving conflicts informally or in a formal way

6.5   Grievances/complaints policy and procedures

6.5.1   Grievance/complaints policy

A grievance or complaint is a dissatisfaction with anything or anyone in the organisation who is thought to be inconsiderate, unjust or unfair.

6.5.2   Aim and purpose of grievance/complaints procedure

The grievance/complaints procedure is designed to be structured in a fair way for an employee to seek to resolve workplace problems. The aim of this procedure is to settle grievances or complaints as near as possible to the point of origin. The procedure is based on the Code of Practice on Disciplinary and Grievances Procedures produced by the Advisory, Conciliation and Arbitration Service (ACAS). Organisations believe that employees should use the established grievance/complaints procedure freely so that management may be assisted in identifying sources of dissatisfaction, and hopefully eliminate them.

6.5.3   Informal and formal procedure

Grievances are frequently caused by misunderstanding. The procedure has two parts: an informal and formal procedure. Informal procedure is where staff takes responsibility of resolving disputes between them as soon as they arise before they escalate. However, there may be occasions where informal approach does not work, or may not be appropriate. In such cases, the employee should raise a formal grievance or complaint.

6.5.4   Formal grievance/complaints procedure

Step 1

The aggrieved employee, be it a regular or Agency staff member, should talk to the project manager and explain their grievance or complaint. If the manager is able to resolve the grievance immediately, s/he is supposed to report back within one week. If after the discussion with the manager it is felt the matter has not been satisfactorily resolved, the person concerned should proceed to step 2.

Step 2

At this stage the grievance or complaint should be discussed with the senior manager who is obliged to report back normally within one week. If the matter is unable to be resolved, and it is wished to proceed further, then the employee should go to step 3.

Step 3

At this stage the employee should formally request, in writing, that his/her grievance or complaint be considered by the senior organisation management (managing director). The written request does not need to have a detailed account of the grievance/complaint. The employee should be given the opportunity to discuss the entire grievance/complaint, together with any results.

Because the managing director has full responsibility for the organisation's operations, his/her decision must be regarded as final and binding.

Important notes to remember

- At no time does the grievance or complaint have to be stated in writing.
- No employee should be reprimanded or made to suffer harassment or victimised from anyone within the organisation as a result of seeking resolution of a grievance or complaint through this procedure.
- An employee may invite a colleague to accompany them as their spokesperson or to assist at any step in the procedure.
- Grievances or complaints which arise from implementation of the disciplinary procedures should be handled by this procedure.
- At any time during the procedure the employee may be asked to attend a meeting to discuss the grievance or complaint in more detail in order to assist in the decision-making process. (If an employee is from an agency, the request for the employee to attend should be made through their agency.)
- Organisations should respect the rights of all individuals to feel comfortable in their working/living environment without fear of being picked on or being bullied.

6.6   Working alone policy

This policy refers to all staff – regular, temporary, agency and volunteer workers in the course of employment. Organisations recognise that some individual workers will be expected to work alone, either at schemes or in the community.

1. All lone workers should have their jobs assessed as part of a risk assessment under the health and safety and Violence at Work Policies.
2. Every scheme/project/place of work where lone working occurs should have a written procedure and guidance of lone working.

3. Written procedures should include the procedure to be adapted in the event that the staff member fails to make contact at an agreed time; the procedure for updating of risk information and the passing on of this information to the relevant parties.

4. In the event of a female staff member becoming pregnant, she should inform her employer/agency and will be risk assessed to indicate whether lone working elements of her duties should be continued.

5. It is the responsibility of lone working staff to ensure safety devices or mobile phones are in proper working condition and to report any concerns, problems or near misses to the managers.

6. It is the responsibility of all staff who are alone and working away from an office base to observe safe practices and not put themselves at risk from any attack or assault.

7. When keeping appointments in the community, staff should ensure that they have a written record for other staff information including the following:

    - where they are going;
    - the name of the person they are visiting;
    - the telephone number of the person they are visiting if available;
    - the expected time of return and duration of the visit.

    Note: If there are any changes to any of the above you should notify your colleagues and the Response Team.

8. All project managers should ensure that an adequate handover system is in place in order that all relevant information is passed on to safeguard the lone worker.

9. All the project/scheme managers responsible for staff, who work alone, should ensure that appropriate safety procedures are in place. This should include the use of personal alarms, automatic warning devices e.g. panic alarms, mobile phones or/and a means of checking in with the response team or sister projects.

10. In the case of an emergency, the lone worker should adhere to the procedure laid down for the scheme/project/place of work, e.g. calling police when faced with violence, or ambulance in a medical emergency

11. Staff should never hesitate to call the police when concerned about their own safety or if they are a victim of a violent incident.

12. Staff who are being asked to lone work, and feel their managers are not taking action to address outstanding risk assessment, should invoke the grievances/complaints procedure.

6.7   Record-keeping policy and procedure

The record keeping policy set out the guideline for report writing and daily entries.

- Always:
    o   write the date;
    o   write the time;
    o   sign each entry;
    o   make entries in black ink, which will makes photocopies clearer, if they are required;

- Entries in the daily diaries should be a factual account of each person's day and should include any extraordinary events or incidents that have occurred. They should be written legibly and indelibly and be clear and unambiguous.
- Avoid using 'fuzzy' descriptions. For example, s/he was aggressive/anxious/happy/in a mood. This kind of record entry is open to personal interpretation. Instead try and describe what the person behaved like. For example, s/he paced backwards and forward briskly, vocalising loudly and swearing loudly.
- Records should not include abbreviations and offensive subjective statements.
- If an event (accident/incident) happens that requires an entry in the Accident/Incident book or an 'ABC' chart, write a concise account in the daily entry and then refer the reader to the appropriate book/chart by writing 'see ABC' or 'accident book'. Write in the daily diary as soon as possible after the event; do not leave it until the end of the shift as you may forget the sequence of events.
- If the service user has an appointment with a health professional, state the date, time and who they saw, refer to the GP's records as above. The GP may be asked to fill in their details in the file as well.
- Never deface records or tear pages out.
- Never use Tippex. If you make a mistake, put a single line through the entry, initial it and continue writing.
- Only the name of the service user may be written in full in service user's file. Staff initials may be used.

6.8   Harassment policy and procedure

6.8.1   What is harassment?

Harassment can take many forms, including racial, or sexual harassment – which may include:

- requests for sexual favours in exchange for promotion, pay rise, or job security;
- touching, pinching or hugging;
- comments, teasing or jokes of a sexual nature;
- staring, winking or leering.

It can range from extreme forms such as violence, to less obvious actions like ignoring someone at work. Whatever the form of harassment, it is unwanted, unreasonable behaviour, which is unwelcome and unpleasant and which the perpetrator knows or should know is offensive, e.g.

- physical contact ranging from touching to serious assault;
- verbal or written harassment through jokes, offensive language, gossip and slander, sectarian songs and letters;
- visual display of posters, graffiti, obscene gestures, flags, bunting and emblems;
- isolation or non-cooperation at work, exclusion from social activities etc.;
- coercion ranging from pressure for sexual favours to pressure to participate in political/religious groups;

- intrusion by pestering, spying, and stalking.

These types of behaviour can cause humiliation, offence, and interference with an individual's work or create an unpleasant, intimidating or hostile working environment.

Some forms of harassment (e.g. sexual and racial) are forms of unlawful discrimination contrary to the Sex Discrimination Act 1975 and the Race Discrimination Act 1976.

6.8.2 Procedure

Harassment has legal implications under the Employment Protection (Consolidation) Act 1978. It is inappropriate behaviour which lowers morale and interferes with work effectiveness.

Ensuring that bullying and harassment does not occur in a workplace requires all employees to be sensitive to the feelings of others and treat them with respect at all times. All organisations regardless of their business, supports the rights and opportunities of all people to obtain and hold employment without discrimination.

Note: If you believe you are being bullied or harassed at work, you should in the first instance make this plain to the perpetrators and ask them to stop the offending behaviour immediately. If the behaviour does not cease, you should make a formal complaint through the organisation's grievances/complaints procedure.

6.9   Confidentiality and privacy policy

6.9.1   Policy aims

The primary aim of this policy is to protect and promote the right to confidentiality and privacy of individual service users, staff members and others with regards to processing and disclosure of personal information.

This policy applies to all personal information held by an organisation in respect to board and committee members, staff, people on placements, volunteers, contractors, service users, potential service users, and applicants for employment, landlords and others.

The secondary aim of confidentiality and privacy policy is to protect commercially sensitive information from unauthorised possession or use.

Organisations must have due regard to the law in protecting the rights of individuals – primarily the Data Protection Act 1998 but also the Human Rights Act 1998 (Article 8), Public Interest Disclosure Act 1998, Crime and Disorder Act 1998, Local Government Act 2000, and Social Security Fraud Act 2001, as amended.

In order to protect the confidentiality and privacy of service users, organisations should require by means of a contract or written agreement any individual or organisations delivering services on its behalf to:

- comply with the law regarding the protection and disclosure of personal information
- not to disclose personal information without a prior written consent of the persons concerned.
- not to attempt to gain personal or commercially sensitive information they are not authorised to have
- keep personal and commercially sensitive information securely whilst in their possession.

6.9.2 Personal data

Personal data is information relating to an individual from whom they can be identified, e.g. name, address, tax details or national insurance number, ethnic origin, health status, income support needs, tenancy history etc., which is held on file, electronically and /or in hard copy. Processing this information is subject to the Data Protection Act 1998.

6.9.3 Commercially sensitive information

Commercially sensitive information is non-personal information about the organisation, its objectives or activities which is intended solely for internal use, because its release could give unfair advantage to external organisations and competitors.

6.9.4 Data Protection Act 1998

The Data Protection Act 1998 states that all personal information held about individuals that is not a matter of public record should be:

- obtained fairly and lawfully;
- held for clear purposes and used only for those purposes;
- relevant, adequate and not excessive;
- accurate, unbiased and kept up-to-date;
- corrected if shown to be inaccurate;
- kept no longer than necessary and destroyed when no longer required;
- protected from loss or disclosure;
- kept secure and treated as confidential at all times.

All staff, volunteers and others engaged in the delivery of services on behalf of the organisation should:

- comply with the law regarding the protection and disclosure of personal information;
- not disclose personal information without prior written informed consent of the person concerned;
- keep personal and commercially sensitive information securely whilst in their possession;
- not attempt to gain personal or commercially sensitive information to which they are not authorised;
- observe any scheme/project/place of work procedures directing where and how personal data should be stored.

Confidentiality must be maintained where personal or commercially sensitive information is in transit or away from the office. In these situations staff should:

- ideally secure confidential data in a bag when on foot;
- lock confidential data in the boot of the car and not leave it in the vehicle overnight.

6.10   Equality and diversity policy

This policy is produced to assist those responsible for recruiting to ensure the organisations are committed to equal opportunities.

- The aim of this policy is to ensure that no job applicant receives less favourable treatment on the grounds of sex, disability, marital status, nationality, colour, religion, ethnic origin, sexual orientation or age.
- Organisations should strive to offer the highest quality service and to ensure the welfare and safety of the service users, clients and colleagues, by recruiting the correct and highest calibre individuals possible for each vacant position. This approach in turn benefits the long-term stability and growth of an organisation and continuity of care.
- Organisations have their own recruitment procedures but always have to follow the action laid down in that procedure.
- Where candidates identify themselves as disabled under the Disability Discrimination Act (DDA), then as long as the individual meets the basic criteria of the job's specification, they should be invited for the interview.
  Organisations should actively seek to recruit staff from all ethnic backgrounds in order to reflect the diversity of their service user groups and offer a full range of practical and interpersonal skills.

6.11   Health and safety policies and procedures

1. Organisations recognise their health and safety duties under the Health and Safety at Work Act 1974 and the Management of Health and Safety at Work Regulations of 1999 and related legislation including the Environmental Protection Act 1990 and the Fire Precautions Act 1971 both as an employer and as an organisation.

2. In recognition of their duties under the Reporting of Injuries, Diseases and Dangerous Occurrences Regulations 1995 (RIDDOR) the organisations should have instituted systems for reporting accidents, diseases and dangerous occurrences to Health and Safety Executive (HSE), including injury to a trainee or agency staff, and this is in addition to its statutory duty to keep an accident book available for inspection by Health and Safety Executive (HSE) inspectors.

3. In furtherance of paragraph 1 the company should propose always to comply with its duties under section 2 of HASAWA 1974 and the Management of Health and Safety at Work Regulations 1999, Regulations 3–7, towards its employees, and more particularly, as far as reasonably practical to:

   - provide and maintain a safe place of work, a safe system of work, safe appliances for work and safe and healthy working environment;
   - provide such information, instructions as may be necessary to ensure the health and safety at work of its employees and also compliance with the Health and Safety Information for Employees Regulations 1989, the Personal Protective Equipment Regulations 1992, the Provision and Use of Work Equipment Regulations 1998, the

Workplace (Health, Safety, and Welfare) Regulations 1992, the Lifting Operations and Lifting Equipment Regulations 1998, the Management of Health and Safety at Work Regulations 1999 and to promote awareness and understanding of health and safety throughout the workforce;

- ensure safety and absence of health risk in conjunction with use, storage and transport of articles and substances;
- make regular risk assessments of employees;
- take appropriate/protective measures;
- where necessary, provide employees with health surveillance;
- appoint competent personnel to secure compliance with the statutory duties.

4. In further recognition of its statutory duty the Company has to take out insurance with an approved insurer against liability for death, injury and/or disease suffered by any of its employees and arising out of and in the course of employment, provided only that it was caused by negligence and/or breach of statutory duty on the part of the company, such certificate of insurance being prominently displayed so as to be available for inspection at all reasonable times by employees or health and safety inspectors.

5. All employees of the company agree, as a term of their contract of employment, to comply with their individual duties under Section 7 of Health and Safety at Work Act 1974, Regulation 14 of the Management of Health and Safety at Work Regulations 1999, and generally cooperate with their employer so as to enable the employer to carry out the health and safety duties towards them. Failure to comply with the health and safety duties, regulations, work rules and procedures relating to health and safety on the part of any employee should lead to dismissal from employment; in case of serious breaches or repeated breaches such dismissal should be instant without prior warning.

6. Prime responsibility for health and safety lies with the managing director of a company and board of directors and the company regards itself as bound by any acts and/or omissions of the managing director, any executive director or senior manager, giving rise to liability, provided only that such acts and or omissions rise out of, and in the course of, company business and prosecution of any director or senior manager, shall not prevent a further prosecution against the company.

6.12   Learning outcomes

- To be able to comply with relevant national legislation or guidance and local policies.
- To be able to recognise workplace hazards and risks.
- To be able to understand and promote safe working practices.
- To understand the importance of acting in ways that are consistent with legislation, policies and procedures for maintaining own and others' health safety and welfare.
- To know how to identify and report any issues at work that may put health, safety and welfare at risk.
- To be able to identify and assess the potential risks involved in work activities and processes for self and others.

6.13   Framework for reflective practice

- ➢ *Knowledge:*   What have you learnt from reading this chapter?
- ➢ *Skills:*   What do you know, or can do differently now, that you did not/could not do before reading this chapter?
- ➢ *Practices:*   How can you perform a task now better than before?

6.14   References

Commission for Social Care Inspection (CSCI): www.csci.org.uk

Department of Health (2002) *Independent Health Care National Minimum Standards Regulations. Patient Confidentiality Standard M3.* London: DoH.

General Social Care Council (2002) *Codes of Practice.* London: GSCC.

Health and Safety Executive (1997) *An Introduction to Health and Safety*, INDG 259. London: HSE.

Health and Safety Executive (2012) *Essentials of Health and Safety at Work*, 4th edn. London: HSE

Social Care Institute for Excellence (SCIE) www.scie.org.uk

6.15   Induction workbook

1. Identify three issues of health and safety legislation relevant to your work setting.

   _____
   _____

2. Summarise your responsibilities in terms of health and safety.

   _____
   _____

3. Give three health and safety responsibilities of a manager in a care setting.

   _____
   _____

4. What health and safety responsibilities do service users have?

   _____
   _____

5. Name two tasks you should not carry out without specialist health and safety training.

   _____
   _____

6. How would you promote safety?

   _____
   _____

7. What is a policy?

    _____

    _____

8. What is a procedure?

    _____

    _____

9. Why is it so important to follow the organisation's policies and procedures?

    _____

    _____

10. List the policies and procedures important for you to know in order to carry out your role properly and safely. Outline the general content of these policies.

    _____

    _____

11. Give a brief summary of the Health and Safety Policy

    _____

    _____

12. How would you involve the service users in your organisation to participate in health and safety?

    _____

    _____

7 The Principles of Support

AIMS

➢ To explain organisations' care planning process and relate this to the requirements of the commissioning body in your work setting

➢ To understand what personalised care planning is

➢ To understand what care plans are and their importance

➢ To understand how care plans may be used to offer holistic support on individualised basis

➢ To identify the difference between a service plan, individual support plan and a care plan

7.1 Care provision

Service users receive a comprehensive assessment of their needs and capabilities. They receive what is termed holistic assessment which means that they are viewed as a whole person who is living with learning disability. The assessment, therefore, considers physical, social, emotional, psychological and educational needs for each individual.

From this assessment a comprehensive plan of care is devised which involves a number of staff members providing different facets of care and a personalised, tailor-made care plan is formulated.

7.2 What is personalised care planning?

Personalised care planning is essentially about addressing an individual's full range of needs, taking into account their health, personal, social, economic, educational, mental health, ethnic and cultural background circumstances. It recognises that there are other issues in addition to medical needs that can impact on a person's total health and well-being. (Dept of Health)

7.3 Care plan

7.3.1 What is a care plan?

A care plan is a structured, often multidisciplinary, task-oriented scheme, detailing the essential steps in the individual care of a service user and describing the expected course of their expected treatment and care. The care plan involves the translation of the needs, strength and risks identified into a written document that is responsive to the phase of the client journey. The care plan should include:

- service user's name;
- key worker's name;
- identified goals in relation to specific support planned.

119

7.3.2   What is care planning?

Care planning is the process of setting goals and interventions based on the needs identified by an assessment and then planning how to meet those goals with the service user. Care planning is a core requirement of structured support

7.3.3   What is a service care plan?

The service care plan is devised when a service user moves into a care setting upon which support is made available and discussed and developed into an agreed service user care plan.

The care plan will include discussions and assessment of risks that the service user or staff may be exposed to as a result of the individual being able to make their own choices and decisions.

This care plan will include:

- discussions and agreement of the service user about who may be involved with the person's care needs;
- care planning;
- any required medications;
- therapies or interventions;
- any aims and goals to be achieved through the implementation of the individual's service care plan.

7.4   Features of a care plan

- Each service user has an individual care plan, which provides the basis on which care and support services should be delivered, with details of how staff help and support the service user to improve their own abilities in everyday life skills.
- Each care plan looks at the level of oral communication understanding and looks at the alternative mode to communicate, e.g. Makaton, Signing, TEACCH, SPELL and symbols-widgit.
- Each person's care plan includes a description of their preferred daily routine, their likes and dislikes and any specific dietary requirement or similar matters.
- It includes their preferences on how they would like to be addressed and what dignity, respect and privacy means to them in terms of daily behaviour and actions.
- The care plan also contains risk assessments and any risk management plans.
- The care plan includes details of individual health care needs, medication, details of their GP, community nursing or other therapeutic or day care services provided.
- The service care plan also includes details of the service user's social interests and activities and how these would be met and any arrangements to attend religious services of their choice or for contact with relatives, friends and representatives or the general community.
- The care plan is also devised to involve a service user in taking an active role in planning of menus and, where possible, in the preparation of meals.

- The service user, with the support of their key worker and staff members, carries out the usual domestic chores of maintaining the cleanliness of their own rooms/flats and communal areas.
- As part of service users' individual day care programmes, many service users access colleges, sports facilities and amenities and have as varied a programme as possible.
- Holidays are organised in either small groups or on an individual basis, depending upon service user's needs and availability of appropriate funding.
- Each individual's day care programme is organised as a response to the service user's individual and combined needs.
- Each service user is allocated a member of the care staff to act as their key worker, who is their named key point of contact. This system enables a service user and staff to build an effective rapport and a relationship of trust, beneficial to the care and development of the service user.

7.5 The role of the key worker in care plan implementation

- Key workers are responsible for monitoring, reviewing and coordinating each service user's individual service care plan.
- Key workers prepare service users' care plans and gather information for their reviews, which are held at least six months or more often if required.
- Key workers are offered regular supervision by their line managers who share responsibility for chairing reviews and for communicating with outside professionals who may be involved with particular service users to ensure that their general needs are met, as well as additional requirements in terms of purchasing clothing, arranging holidays, visits to the doctors/dentist etc.
- The key worker should liaise and collaborate with other providers to coordinate care. This may include referral, liaison or joint working towards goals with other service providers and tracking client progress across a range of providers.

7.6 Individual support plans

Individual support plans sets out the kind of support a service user needs and helps them and their support worker to see if they are making progress.

- Some of the targets in the support plan are short term, such as getting a qualification and work placement.
- The key worker draws a support plan within two weeks of a service user moving into a care setting.
- The support plans are reviewed regularly to assess progress and ensure they are still meeting the needs of the service user.

7.7 What is in the individual support plan?

The support plan is divided into three sections:

1. issues

2. aims
3. actions

- The *issues* section is used to identify service users' needs.
- The *aims* section is used to identify the outcome they want.
- The *actions* section sets out the steps that the service user needs to work through in order to achieve their goals.

7.8   Person-centred plans

- Person-centred planning provides a way to consider important developments in people's lives as part of a regular overall review of what has been achieved and what might be possible in the future.
- In person-centred planning, individual preferences and the involvement of the person concerned in deciding what outcomes to pursue are essential.
- In person-centred plans, objectives may be agreed for developing a person's activities, social relationships, learning, independence, autonomy, health, job placement, home or some other aspect important to his/her quality life.
- The objectives then need to be translated into action and taken forward; this can be achieved through active support which is complementary

7.9   What are the important things in supporting people?

For the *people being supported* the important things are:

- staff consistency;
- having a laugh and fun;
- creating a pleasant and respectful welcoming environment;
- being safe;
- being supported to do what they want;
- having choice;
- knowing routines;
- being understood;
- trust;
- being warm and cosy;
- having good health food;
- being treated and accorded respect;
- people being kind, compassionate, caring and having empathy.

For the *families* the important things are:

- honesty;
- making people we support happy;
- good quality of staff;
- consistency;

- open dialogue;
- safety;
- trust;
- keeping people we support active, healthy and happy;
- creating a pleasant and respectful welcoming environment;
- making a house a home.

For the *support teams* the important things are:

- consistency;
- enduring;
- getting support;
- flexibility;
- good staff team and trust;
- being committed;
- good personal philosophy;
- caring;
- trust.

For *Social Services/Care Quality Commission* the important things are:

- reliability of staff
- evidence of safety
- safeguarding
- staff training
- being honest and open

7.10   Active support

Jones *et al.* (2011) say that active support helps people lead full lives, and is designed to make sure that people who need support have the chance to be fully involved in their lives and receive the right range and level of support to be successful.

Active support has three components:

1. interacting to promote participation;
2. activity support plans;
3. keeping tracks.

7.10.1   Principles of active support

Although every one of us differs, there are some core elements we all have in common. It is important for most people to:

- be part of a community;
- have good relationships with friends and family;

- have relationships that last;
- have opportunities to develop experience and learn new skills;
- have choices and control over life;
- be afforded status and respect; and
- be treated as an individual

These core elements of life have come to define what we mean by leading a socially valued lifestyle which can be achieved through active support.

7.10.2 Where active support fits in

Active support is used alongside other approaches that are designed to achieve other aims, such as:

- person-centred plans;
- opportunity or learning plans;
- positive behavioural support;
- communication plans.

7.10.3 Why is active support important?

Providing support bridges the gap between what people can and cannot do. Active support outlines how to assist people effectively and to structure activities so that the steps match the individual's abilities.

Active support helps us:

- keep fit and mentally alert;
- express who we are;
- establish common interest with others; we connect with others by appealing to the similarities we all share;
- provide the basis for friendships and for living together;
- develop our talents and show what we can do;
- and is the means by which we look after ourselves and our daily needs.

7.10.4 Support and planning

Good support can help fill the gap for people with learning disabilities to participate in activities. This means planning for the best use of time and giving them as much support as they need to get things done for themselves. The greater the severity of disability the larger the knowledge or skills gap becomes. With sufficient planning and support, everybody can:

- participate in activities and have a full day regardless of their disability;
- contribute if they haven't got all the skills needed for a particular activity;
- take on their share of responsibility; and
- be involved in things they like to do or make informed choices.

Planning is a way of supporting people; it shows commitment.

Most of us have a good idea of what we are going to do each day. We all make use of plans, even if they are only in our heads. We have basic routines, we think about what we have to do each day and then what we would like to do, we make lists; we make appointments and keep diaries.

We often feel like we have got too much to do, so we have plans regarding how to fit it all in. People with learning disabilities often have too little to do. They spend time waiting, perhaps bored, for the next opportunity to do something and make a contribution. Planning for a full day can help people lead more fulfilling lives.

Things to remember about the people being supported:

- Every individual has strengths, gifts and contributions to offer.
- Every individual has the ability to express preferences and to make choice given the right support.
- Every individual has hopes, dreams and desires.
- Don't rely on service user's memory. Use visual aids to enhance memory such as calendars, visual timetables, object of reference and other memory aides. Visual memory tends to be better than auditory memory. It's easier to remember what we see than what we hear. Use both at the same time to enhance memory.
- Routine: Maintain routines, like taking medications at the same time every day.
- Associate stories with new things or ideas.
- Allow additional time and have patience.

7.10.5 How to support engagement

The goal of active engagement
By supporting individuals you can help them engage in managing their own lives and in pursuing their interests and hobbies.

Matching support to need
The level of support provided is matched directly to the individual's abilities and need for support in each activity, always making it person-centred in practice. While the support provided has to be adequate, the aim is always to promote independence by giving only as much support as is needed. Assistance is gradually minimised as practice makes the person more competent.

7.10.6 Ways of giving support

Different types of support give more or less help. For example, telling somebody how to use a toaster. We can think of the different levels of support in the following order:

ASK – INSTRUCT – PROMPT – SHOW – GUIDE

- **ASK** – (SUGGEST or TELL) is a verbal prompt which lets someone know it is time to do something or that something needs to be done. For example, running a bath
  ASK may be all the support a person needs if they can basically do the activity.

- **INSTRUCT** is a series of verbal prompts which tell the individual what to do one step at a time. It helps to guide an individual through the activity. For example: having a bath.

  INSTRUCT works well when an individual can physically do the task but needs to be reminded of the sequence of steps. It also depends on an individual's ability to understand instructions. Using simple clear directions is most helpful

- **PROMPT** is a clear gesture or sign to tell an individual what to do next. Briefly mimic an act, e.g. dressing. PROMPT works better by miming an act which can provide a lot of information for the individual to follow, especially when the individual does not easily understand words but is able to interpret and follow gestures or respond to signs of what to do next.

- **SHOW** is demonstrating what needs to be done. A demonstration is more definite and provides more information than a prompt. It provides a higher level of support. Your role is to give a demonstration and then the individual follows and does the same thing immediately afterwards. SHOW can be combined with PROMPT or INSTRUCT.

  SHOW works well when an individual does not know what to do but is able to imitate.

- **GUIDE** is giving an individual direct physical assistance to do something. This type of physical support and how long is done vary according to an individual's need for support. Placing your hand over the individual's hand and guiding it gives more support than guidance at the wrist or forearm. Guidance may be given only at the beginning of a step to get the individual started (like prompt), or it may be given throughout the steps. GUIDE can be combined with PROMPT or INSTRUCT and can follow SHOW.

  Example: Guiding an individual's hand at the wrist when supporting them to brush their teeth.

  GUIDE works well when an individual needs a lot of support. Make notes of order in which different parts of an activity is done. For example, brushing teeth.

7.10.7 Thinking in steps

Most activities are a sequence of steps. Guidance for activities is often set out in a series of steps as in a recipe book or a DIY manual. Being aware of the sequence of steps within an activity is useful when supporting people with learning disabilities to participate or learn new skills, making notes of order in which different parts of an activity is done. The process of breaking an activity into small steps is sometimes called task analysis.

Thinking in small steps is particularly helpful for people with more severe learning disabilities. Each step can then be supported at an appropriate level using ASK – INSTRUCT - PROMPT – SHOW – GUIDE.

The degree to which you break a task down can vary from a few steps to many smaller steps. Support can lessen and the number of steps reduced as people get better at an activity.

7.10.8 Feedback

Performance feedback: The value of activities is something everyone has to learn. People need recognition for what they achieve and need encouragement along the way. Here praise is important. Praise is a gift that costs the giver nothing but is priceless to the recipient. Praise helps people to recognise that they are doing something useful and doing it well.

For more details on active support, see: **http//arcuk.org.uk...ppot-Handbook.pdf**

7.11   Tools of support

- A person with autism functions best with literal, concrete terms and not abstractly, which means explaining a concept with detailed descriptions is not as effective as showing pictures (visual) or the object itself.
- The individual may also have trouble transferring a freshly learned skill, but using visual symbols should help the individual to think conceptually by guiding them to put details together to form ideas through use of the TEACCH approach.

7.12   TEACCH

TEACCH stands for Treatment and Education of Autistic and Communication Handicapped Children. It is recognised as an outstanding programme by the American Psychiatric Association, the National Institute of Mental Health and the American Psychological Association.

7.12.1   What is TEACCH?

TEACCH development began in the 1970 as a reaction against the prevailing thoughts that autism is an emotional disorder. TEACCH is more of philosophy of treatment rather than an intervention – a philosophy based on assessing children with autism for their needs and using already existing approaches to help them lead fulfilling and productive lives.

- TEACCH focuses on tailoring individualised programmes, building on existing skills, interests and respecting the 'culture of autism'.
- TEACCH emphasises building on strengths more than remedying weaknesses.
- TEACCH emphasises understanding the characteristics of people with autism as a basis for arranging their environments to maximise success.

7.12.2   Understanding how TEACCH works

According to Mesibov *et al.* (2005) practitioners employ the following elements to ensure that the structured-teaching approach works with the characteristics of people with autism spectrum disorders.

7.12.3   Organisation of physical environment

- Children/adults with ASD don't always understand where they are suppose to start; therefore, clear physical boundaries can help using TEACCH, whether at school, home, the workplace or in the community.
- The boundaries are made clear through placement of furniture and through visual cues such as words for those individuals who can read and pictorial reminders for those children who cannot read. For example, in the garden centre, boundaries are set in one corner using chairs and a table to mark a place for coffee breaks.

7.12.4 Predictable sequence of events

- Predictability is important for reducing anxiety and helping people with autism become productive and successful.
- Predictability can be achieved by implementing a daily schedule or a pre-planned series of steps for activities such as in the shower/bath times, work projects, therapy sessions, house chores and recreation.
- TEACCH provides a 'to do list' for people with autism, which include setting for both a regular class/activity schedule and an individual schedule for personal activities.

7.12.5 Routines with flexibility

- Routines can help provide a sense of order and predictability in a confusing world for people with autism and to support them to be prepared for a world of continual changes. However, in order to prevent people with autism from developing non-functional routines such as having to smell all computers keyboards in a computer lab prior to starting work, prescribing health routines helps.
- Flexibility should be built into routines, for example routines for medication structure can be maintained at the same time but changes can be made in variations in food, clothes they wear, different route to town or taking public means of transport etc.

7.13 Visual schedules

People with autism have a tendency to be visually based rather than language based, therefore it is important to provide a picture or written schedule for reference, which help reduce the possibility of a person forgetting what have been previously communicated orally.

- A visual schedule can also help through transition such as getting on the bus to start a school day, end of a school semester or end of an activity or using public transport.
- A visual schedule fosters independence from adult support later in life in addition to promoting feelings of security and competence.
- Visual schedules can be text-based for people able to read or pictorial for people who have not yet developed reading skills.
- To reinforce visual schedules, objects of reference may be used such as a plate to represent lunch/dinner time, or a mouse to represent computer time.

TEACCH practitioners emphasise the importance of making sure that each day's schedule (timetables) varies from the previous day to some extent in order to keep the children/adult with autism from getting too attached to a routine.

See above, Figure 2.2, p. 64, for an example of a structured visual timetable.

7.13.1 Visually structured activities and work systems

Many children and adults on the autism disorder spectrum have poor auditory processing skills and tend to have considerable visual strength combined with a need for tangible representation of tasks or activities. In order to engage interest in an individual with autism more successfully, they will need something to see, touch, or hold.

The task to an individual with autism, using TEACCH, will include the following:

- *Instructions*: Visual instructions work when a person can physically do the task but needs to be reminded of the sequence of steps. It does also depend on the person's ability to understand the instructions. Using simple, clear directions is most helpful.
- *Clarity*: Providing too many objects for a task can confuse people with ASD. However, objects can be grouped into categories, usually for some specific purpose. The ideas and objects are recognised, differentiated, and understood by using different shapes, colour and textures to accentuate the differences.
- *Organisation*: Many people with autism become overwhelmed when objects are in disorder, perhaps some objects are covering others so they cannot be seen; it is important that objects are organised in order before the individual being supported with an activity begins working with them.

7.13.2 Structured work systems

Structured work systems offer a tool for assisting individuals with ASD to focus on important details, maintaining attention to tasks, and generalising skills learned in one setting to new environments, which provide a meaningful way to approach activities and situations, indicating the passage of time between the beginning, middle and the end of an activity.

The work systems approach the organisation of an activity with the following four elements in mind:

- What activities to complete? This describes the activities or task. For example, filling flower pots with soil in a garden centre.
- How many activities to complete? In other words, quantity. In this case how many flowerpots will the individual fill?
- When am I finished? Measuring progress is usually done visually. The staff can use a timer or the decreasing number of flowerpots left to be filled with soil, which can serve as a visual stats cue. The end of an activity can be signified by a short break to celebrate.
- What happens next? For the flower filling pots with soil task, staff can signify the completion of the task by washing of hands indicating the next step. The next steps may include giving a reward or taking a lunch break or going home.

7.13.3 Summary of structured work systems

As with schedules, structured work systems can be represented in a way the individual can understand – be it with words, pictures, or objects for individuals who are nonverbal or for those who have not yet developed reading skills.

- Offer a clear and predictable sequence of activities to complete. Such predictability helps to decrease anxiety and uncertainty that many individuals with ASD feel in the face of unfamiliar/new tasks or activities.
- Promote independence and limit the need for constant adult support and prompting and the need for verbal instructions.

- Provide an external organisation tool for individuals with ASD who may have trouble organising objects.
- Reduce and help limit distractions by grouping and highlighting the important information in an activity.
- Once an individual has learned how to use it, the system can be used across environments to promote generalisation of skills and offer choices.

7.13.4 Example of visually structured activity

Washing hands

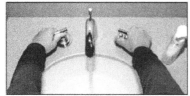
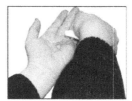

1. Turn on the water.   2. Put soap on your hands.   3. Lather.

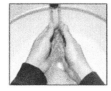
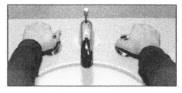
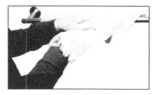

4. Rinse.   5. Turn off the water.   6. Dry hands.

7.14   Learning outcomes

- To help deliver other cross-government strategies, including Valuing People Now and Valuing Employment Now for people with learning disabilities.
- To recognise through Putting People First that person-centred planning and self-directed support are central to delivering personalisation and maximising choice and control.
- To support service users in achieving their aspirations and ambitions and being able to provide access to their communities.
- To support service users in meeting their goals, and promoting cross-cultural sensitivity for all service users.
- To ensure that the personal choices of the people being supported are always held as central to our work and our professional decisions at individual and organisational level.

7.15   Framework for reflective practice

- ➢ *Knowledge:* What have you learnt from reading this chapter?
- ➢ *Skills:* What do you know, or can do differently now, that you did not/could not do before reading this chapter?
- ➢ *Practices:* How can you perform a task now better than before?

7.16   References

Department of Health (2004) *NHS Improvement Plan 2004: Putting People at the Heart of Public Services.* London: DoH.

Department of Health (2004) *Standards for Better Health.* London: DoH.

Hewett, D. and Nind, M. (1998) *Interaction in Action: Reflections on the Use of Intensive Interaction.* London: David Fulton.

Holburn, S. and Vietze, P. (2002) *Person-centred Planning: Research, Practice, and Future Directions.* Baltimore, Maryland: Paul H Brookes.

Jones, E., Perry, J., Lowe, K, Allen, D., Toogood, S. and Felce, D. (2011) *Active Support: Handbook for Supporting People with Learning Disabilities to Lead Full Lives.* ARC Cymru.

Mesibov, G.B., Shea, V. and Shopler, E. (2005) *The TEACCH Approach to Autism Spectrum Disorders.* New York: Springer.

National Health Service (1990) *NHS and Community Care Act 1990.* London: HMSO.

Thompson, N. and Thompson, S. (2008) *The Social Work Companion.* London: Palgrave Macmillan.

Toogood, S. (in press) *Person-centred Action Plans.* Brighton: Pier Publishing.

Wing, L. (2002) The Autistic Spectrum, New Updated Edition. London: Constable & Robinson.

7.17   Induction workbook

1. What is a care plan?

2. What are three ways of making sure you always work in a person-centred way?

3. Describe how and when you should use a risk assessment for a service user.

4. Who might be involved in the risk assessment process?

5. Who should you inform about any risk you have identified and how would you do this?

6. Why is it important that members of the team know what each is doing and work in a coordinated way? What system allows this to happen?

8　Record-keeping

AIMS

- To be able to write entries in daily diaries of service users in accordance with the organisations policies and procedures

- To identify the benefits of effective record keeping and the implications of poor record-keeping

- To explain organisation's care planning process and relate this to the requirements of the Commissioning Body in your work setting

- To relate daily entries in service users' notes to individual care plans

8.1　Introduction

8.1.1　What is record-keeping?

Record-keeping is the practice of maintaining the records of an organisation from the time they are created up to their eventual disposal.

- This may include classifying, storing, securing, and destruction (or in some cases, archival preservation) of records.
- Record-keeping is primarily concerned with the evidence of an organisation's activities, and is usually applied according to the value of the records rather than their physical format.
- A high standard of record-keeping is fundamental to the delivery of safe and professional care.
- The provision of a record-keeping policy provides the framework to guide professional practice in accordance with the Data Protection Act (1998).

8.1.2　Importance of record-keeping

Good-quality record-keeping:

- provides security to both patients and staff, achieved by good-quality record-keeping leading to an accurate record of care, continuity of care, and ensuring high standards of health and social care provision;
- promotes better communication as well as continuity, consistency, and efficiency, and reinforces professionalism within a care environment;
- ensures a consistent approach to service users' support; it shows the chronology of events, the care implementation, responses to care and treatment;
- demonstrates that staff have exercised their accountability and fulfilled their legal and professional duty of care;
- leads to an accurate record of care, continuity of care and decisions made relating to the service users' care;

- facilitates fast retrieval of information, evidence of communication between staff, and dissemination of information;
- ensures that the professional and legal standing of staff are not undermined by absent or incomplete records; records provide tangible evidence, if they are called to account at a hearing in a court of law.

As with all areas of health and social care practice, record-keeping must be audited on a regular basis to ensure compliance with the standards that have been set in accordance with the Data Protection Act (1998), which also incorporates the Access to Health Records Act (1990) and Care Standards Act (2000) and National Minimum Standards Regulations

8.1.3 Scope of record-keeping policy

In record-keeping the terms 'notes' and 'documents' are used frequently in professional practice in health and social care. These terms refer to any record that has a service user's name on it. This, therefore, includes all medical and nursing records and any other records made by members of the organisation staff, diaries as well as letters, correspondences and all electronic formats.

8.2 Guidelines to writing daily notes

- Records are to be factual, consistent, accurate and in chronological order.
- Records should be written as soon as possible after an event has occurred using reflective practice, providing current information on the care/condition of the service user.
- Records should provide clear evidence of the care planned, the decisions made, the care given and the information shared.
- Records should be written in such a manner that any alterations or additions are dated, timed using the 24-hour clock and signed with the author's name printed alongside when making the first entry and include the author's position.
- Records should not include abbreviations, jargon, meaningless phrases, irrelevant speculation and offensive subjective statements.
- Records should be readable on any photocopies.
- Records should be clearly written and legible.

8.2.1 Example of a record entry in a daily diary

```
19.08.09  1400hrs  Shelby  awoke  at  0930hrs.  She  attended
computers  at  the  day  centre  and  Art  and  Craft  in  the
activity  room.  Interacted  well  with  staff  and  fellow
residents,  chatting  and  socialising,  received  a  telephone
call  from  her  sister.  Shelby  stated  she  was  pleased  her
sister called. No evidence of self-harming (Care Plan 2) did
not  display  any  aggression  (Care  Plan  4),  attended  meal,
sitting  and  ate  breakfast  and  lunch  (Care  Plan  3);  attended
personal  care,  needed  some  prompting,  reminded  to  go  for  a
shower  on  two  occasions  before  going  (Care  Plan  1).

G. Jones. Support Worker
```

8.3   Why do we keep daily records?

Good record keeping in a service:

- promotes continuity of care and ensure consistency in support;
- demonstrates high standards of care and evidence of care being given, the intervention by professional practitioners and service users' responses;
- enhances communication and sharing of information between staff and other professionals;
- daily records help to protect service users and staff by keeping accurate records of the action taken and the care given;
- allows deterioration/progress in service users' condition to be detected at an early stage;
- provides the chronology of events and the reasons for any decisions made;
- enables all members of the multidisciplinary team to care for the service user regardless of what stages they have reached in the care process;
- good records can be used in a court of law;
- for monitoring and review purposes.

8.4   Standards for documents

Standards for record-keeping should include:

- When possible, daily records should be written with the involvement of the service user and written in a language that is understandable to them.
- The service user should be read the outline of his/her care plans. They should sign if they have the capacity to do so and should be given a copy. If the service user refuses to sign this must be documented.
- Records should identify problems that have risen and what action has been taken to rectify the problem.
- Daily records should provide evidence of the care planned and this should be acknowledged in progress notes.
- Daily records should show clear evidence of the care planned, the decisions made, the care delivered and the information shared.

8.5   Legislation and documentation policies

- Under the Data Protection Act 1998, patients/service users have the right of access to their manual health records. This must be considered at all times when undertaking records and documentation.
- Patients/service users also have legal rights of access to their computer-held records and all information held on them.
- All service users' records can be required as evidence in a court of law, professional conduct committee and other similar regulatory bodies. This must be considered when undertaking any documentation.

- There are specific requirements regarding record-keeping under the Mental Health Act (1983). The Mental Health Act 1983 Code of Practice makes the following statements in reference to record keeping;

  o With reference to receipt of section papers: The hospital should have a checklist for the guidance of those delegated to receive documents to detect errors that cannot be corrected at a later stage in the procedure.
  o With reference to leave periods (Section 17 of Mental Health Act): The granting of leave and the conditions attached to it should be recorded in the service user's notes and copies given to the service user, any appropriate relatives or friends and any professionals in the community who need to know.
  o With reference to complaints: As a matter of good practice complaints records should be kept separate from health records (see Grievances and complaints policy and procedures, Section 6.5).

8.6   Record-keeping and confidentiality

- Information contained in service users' records should be held in complete *confidence* and viewed only by those directly involved in the care of the service users or authorised personnel.
- The service user can give written consent for release of information to specified individuals. While particular services have their own *confidentiality* policies, consent from the service user may be sought prior to release of information to other professionals.
- When service user information is required for clinical audit it must be presented in anonymous form to protect *confidentiality*. Anonymous form means that any means of identifying the service user is removed.
- The *confidentiality* of other service users must be respected. Therefore confidential or identifiable information must not be entered into any other service users' records. The use of initials may be used.
- *Confidentiality* may be breached if the service user is believed to be at risk to themselves or others or if the organisation is subpoenaed to provide evidence in a court of law.
- The rights to *confidentiality* can be waived if the information regarding a service user is required either by National Health Services (NHS) organisations or by any organisation outside the NHS, for example social services, probation etc., in which case The Caldicott Principles should apply (see Chapter 3, Section 3.11).
- All correspondences from the clinical area containing any information about a service user must be marked private and confidential on the outside of the envelope.

8.7   Consequences of poor record-keeping

8.7.1   Consequences for individuals (service users)

- There could be allegations of criminal activity without defence.
- No evidence of care provision and lack of continuity of care.
- Never shows records of progress or deterioration or reviews.
- Only bad things are written.

8.7.2 Consequences for staff and organisation

- Inconsistency through bad communication.
- The organisation can fail inspection.
- Allegations of staff not being competent and/or abusive.
- Lack of documented evidence of the care planned and progress made by the service user.
- Lack of evidence of continuity of care to the service user.
- Lack of facilitated fast retrieval of information and failure to comply with the standards that have been set.

8.8 When access to information should be denied

When a service user requests access to any data held on them, the request must be made in writing to the hospital manager or the care setting they are supported in and no reason needs to be given. The applicant must be given a copy of the information and if appropriate an explanation.

In the following exceptional circumstances information may be withheld:

- where permitting access to the data would be likely to cause serious harm to the physical condition of the data subject or any other person (which may include a health care professional);
- where disclosing the data would reveal information which relates to and identifies another person, unless that person has consented to the disclosure;
- if the request is made by another on behalf of the subject such as a parent for a child, access can be refused if the subject provided the information in the expectation that it would not be disclosed.
- the decision to refuse access to records must be by all professionals involved in the service user's care; the reasons for this decision must be clearly documented in the service user's notes.

8.9 Storage and transportation of records

1. Records must be stored in an area that ensures neither other service users, members of the public, nor unauthorised members of staff can gain access to them.
2. Where records are stored in areas that do not have 24-hour staff presence, then they must be stored in an area that can be securely locked when the premises are unstaffed.
3. If records need to be transported from one organisation to another agency, it is the responsibility of the staff member to ensure that at no point could the records be accessed by unauthorised individuals.
4. It is the staff members' responsibility to ensure that any records are stored safely and securely whilst in transit.

8.10 Computer-held records

- All computer records held or transmitted are subject to the same controls as manually held records under the Data Protection Act 1998.

- If information is to be transmitted by fax or email, the member of staff choosing this method of communication is responsible for ensuring that all information transmitted remains confidential.
- All computer-held records must be password-protected and only accessible by authorised users.

8.11   How to write daily notes

Service users at all residential care homes/supported living/housing projects will have a service user file, in which staff will make a record of service users' daily movements, appointments and incidents. All entries must be written in a respecting and positive manner.

The record-keeping policy sets out the guidelines for report writing and daily entries (see Chapter 6, Section 6.7). Remember to allow yourself plenty of time to make your entries into the service users file; do not leave it until 5 minutes before your shift ends.

Note: Service user files and all other written documentation at residential homes or supported living/housing projects are kept for many years as a legal requirement. They can be used in the event of an inquiry into a project or residential home.

8.12   Learning outcomes

By the end of this chapter, you will be able to:

- write entries in daily diaries of service users in accordance with the organisation's policies and procedures;
- identify the benefits of effective record-keeping and the implications of poor record keeping;
- explain your organisation's care planning process and relate this to the requirements of the commissioning body in your work setting;
- relate daily entries in service users' notes to individual care plans.

8.13   Framework for reflective practice

➢ *Knowledge:*   What have you learnt from reading this chapter?
➢ *Skills:*   What do you know, or can do differently now, that you did not/could not do before reading this chapter?
➢ *Practices:*   How can you perform a task now better than before?

8.14   References

Day-Stirk, F. and Steele, R. (2001) Clinical risk management paper 4: communication and record keeping, *RCM Midwives Journal* **4**(3): 82–3.

Department of Health (1993) A *Vision for the Future: The Nursing Midwifery and Health Visiting Contribution to Health and Healthcare*. HMSO, London

Department of Health (2006) *Records Management: NHS Code of Practice Part 1*.London: DoH.

Department of Health (2009) *Records Management: NHS Code of Practice Part 2*, 2nd edn. London: DoH.

Ghaye, T. and Lillyman, S (2010) *Reflection: Principles and Practice for Healthcare Professionals*. 2nd edn. London: Quay Books.

Hoban, V. (2003) How to improve your record keeping, *Nursing Times* **99**(42):78-9.

Jarvis P (1992) Reflective practice and nursing. *Nurse Education Today* **12**: 174–81.

Jasper, M. (2003) *Beginning Reflective Practice – Foundations in Nursing and Healthcare*. Cheltenham: Nelson Thornes.

Johns, C. (2000) *Becoming a Reflective Practitioner*. Oxford: Blackwell Science.

Nursing and Midwifery Council (2002) *Guidelines for Records and Record Keeping*. London: NMC.

Schon, D. (1983) *The Reflective Practitioner*. London: Basic Books.

Thompson, N. and Thompson, S. (2008) *The Social Work Companion*. London: Palgrave Macmillan.

Tinsley, V. (2002) Record keeping for dummies, *British Journal of Midwifery* **10**(3): 158.

8.15   Induction workbook

1. Explain why it is important to keep full and accurate records.
    _____
    _____

2. Identify four different records that you contribute to, explaining their purpose.
    _____
    _____

3. What is the difference between opinion and fact?
    _____
    _____

4. Explain why it is important to ensure that all records are:

    Factual
    _____
    _____

    Relevant to their purpose
    _____
    _____

    Clear, concise and easy to understand
    _____
    _____

    Signed and dated

9 Discrimination, Equality and Diversity

AIMS

- To raise awareness about diversity
- To inform staff in care settings strategies how to address issues of a diversity nature
- To promote good practice
- To understand the reporting and feedback procedures

9.1 Diversity

Diversity is about creating a working culture that seeks to respect value and harness differences.

- Diversity, rather than judging people and ideas by the extent to which they conform to our existing values, recognises that those differences provide opportunities for a richer, more creative business environment that can better provide for the diverse nature of our service users.
- Diversity is proactive and inclusive, taking in visible differences such as gender, ethnicity and disability, as well as differences that are not necessarily and immediately apparent, such as sexual orientation, religious beliefs and nationality.

9.2 Equality (equal opportunities)

Equal opportunities are about providing fair and equal access/treatment for everybody. In the past, movements aiming for equality's have been seen as reactive, often driven by legal requirement.

Equal opportunities movements have looked at the problems presented by differences between particular groups and sought to prevent discrimination by concentrating on those groups who might face discrimination.

9.2.1 How to implement equal opportunities policy

Organisations should be committed to implement the equal opportunities policy, trusting that every employee should have an individual responsibility. All employees should be required to comply with the policy and act in accordance with its objectives so as to remove any barriers to equal opportunities. There are specific employees' responsibilities which include:

- not inducing or attempting to induce others to practice unlawful discrimination;
- reporting any discriminatory action as soon as is practically possible;
- not discriminating against colleagues, service users, families and friends of service user or members of the public with whom they come into contact during the course of their duties.

9.3   Factors that may lead to social exclusion

Social exclusion means that service users are excluded from joining society through 'factors beyond their control'. These might be issue such as:

- insecure, low paid, low quality employment;
- low levels of education, illiteracy;
- growing up in a vulnerable family (e.g. single parent, domestic violence);
- disability;
- poor health;
- living in a multiple deprivation (crime, drugs, antisocial behaviour);
- homelessness and precarious conditions;
- immigration, ethnicity, racism and discrimination;
- de-institutionalisation (prisons, institutional care, mental institutions);
- age.

9.4   The nine strands of diversity (protected characteristics)

The Equality Act 2010 came into effect in October 2010 and replaced previous anti-discrimination laws with a single act to make the law simpler and to remove inconsistencies. This makes the law easier for people to understand and comply with. The act also strengthened protection in some situations.

 The act covers nine protected characteristics, which cannot be used as a reason to treat people unfairly. Every person has one or more of the protected characteristics, so the act protects everyone against unfair treatment.

9.4.1   Age

Age may be defined as 'the length of time that one has existed; duration of life'.

Key legislation

- Employment Equality (Age) Regulation 2006.

The Employment Equality Regulation from 1 October 2006 made it unlawful to discriminate against workers, employees, job seekers and trainees because of their age. The regulation covers recruitment, terms and conditions, promotions, transfers, termination and training.

- Equality Act 2010

The Equality Act 2010 protects people of all ages. However, different treatment because of age is not unlawful, direct or indirect discrimination if it can be justified, that is if a person can demonstrate that it is a proportionate means of meeting a legitimate aim. Age is the only protected characteristic that allows employers to justify direct discrimination.

9.4.2   Disability

Disability is a physical or mental condition that limits a person's movement, senses or activities. The Disability Discrimination Act (1995) defines disability as 'a physical or mental impairment which has a substantial and long-term adverse effect on a person's ability to carry out normal day-to-day activities'. The definition of disability from the Disability Discrimination Act (DDA) 2005 indicates that there are five main categories of disabilities, which include:

- mobility impairment – moving from place to place;
- sensory impairment – blindness and deafness;
- mental health issues;
- learning difficulties;
- long-term ill health issues (chronic illnesses).

Key legislation

- Disability Equality Duty 2006
- Disability Discrimination Act (DDA) 1995
- Disability Discrimination Act (DDA) 2005

The Disability Discrimination Act (DDA) makes it unlawful to discriminate against disabled people in a number of areas including: employment, access to goods and services, education and transport.

In April 2005 the Act was amended and the definition of disability extended to include: HIV, multiple sclerosis and cancer – on diagnosis.

There was also a change in the classification for mental illness, which no longer needs to be 'clinically' well recognised to be classed as impairment.

The new Legislation introduced in 2006 places:
- a duty on public bodies to actively promote disability equality; some provisions that have helped in this respect are:

  o   improved access or layout by using ramps in public transport;
  o   building wheelchair-friendly layout to access buildings;
  o   using voice prompts in lifts and low positions buttons to access building floors;
  o   producing information in large print and font sizes, audio cd, use of Braille and easy read and Plain English formats in line with its translation procedures.

- a specific duty to publish a Disability Equality Scheme (DES). The scheme should set out how organisations intend to meet the general duty and be reviewed every three years.

- Equality Act 2010

Under the Equality Act, a person is disabled if they have a physical or mental impairment which has substantial and long-term adverse effect on their ability to carry out normal day-to-day activities, which could include things like reading a book, or using public transport or accessing buildings.

The Act puts a duty on the employer to make reasonable adjustments for employees to help them overcome disadvantages resulting from their impairment.

The Act includes protection from discrimination arising from disability. This states that it is discrimination to treat a disabled person unfavourably because of something connected with their disability (e.g. a tendency to make spelling mistakes from being dyslexic). This type of discrimination is unlawful where the employer or their representative knows, or could reasonably be expected to know, that the person has disability.

Moreover, indirect discrimination now covers disabled people. This means that a job applicant or employee could claim that a particular rule or requirement in place disadvantages people with the same disability. Unless it can be justified, it would be unlawful.

The Act also includes a new provision which makes it unlawful, except in certain circumstances, for employers to ask about a candidate's health before offering them employment.

9.4.3   Gender

Gender, as defined by Oxford Dictionary, is 'the state of being male or female (typically used in reference to social and cultural differences rather than biological ones)'.

Key legislation

- The Equality Act 2006 (Gender Equality Duty)
- Sex Discrimination Act 1975
- Equal Pay Act 1970
- The Equality Act 2010

Discrimination by gender has been prohibited by the Sex Discrimination Act 1975, in relation to employment and provision of goods, facilities and services. However, under the Gender Equality Duty, public bodies are required to actively promote gender equality through their key functions.

The duty requires public authorities to have due regard to the need to:

- eliminate unlawful discrimination with regard to obligations under the Sex Discrimination Act 1975 and the Equality Pay Act 1970, and to take steps to ensure compliance with these Acts;
- promote equality of opportunity between men and women, and to take active steps to promote gender equality when carrying out functions and activities, which include specific duties like:

  o publishing gender equality schemes, including equal pay policies, in consultation with employees and stakeholders;
  o monitoring progress and publishing progress reports every three years;
  o conducting and publishing gender impact assessment on major legislation and policy.

9.4.4 Marriage and civil partnership

The Equality Act 2010 protects employees who are married or in civil partnership against discrimination. Single people are not protected.

9.4.5 Pregnancy and maternity

A woman is protected against discrimination on the grounds of pregnancy and maternity. During the period of her pregnancy any statutory leave to which she is entitled during this period. An employer must not take into account an employee's period of absence due to pregnancy related illness when making a decision about her employment. Pregnancy and maternity discrimination cannot be treated as sex discrimination.

9.4.6 Race and ethnicity

Race is used to describe genetic heritage (including one's skin colour, and associated traits) whereas ethnicity describes one's cultural background or allegiance.

Key legislation

- Race Relations Act 1976
- Race Relations (Amendment) Act 2000
- Equality Act 2010

Under the general duty of the Race Relations (Amendment) Act 2000, employers are required to promote race equality with due regard to the need to:

- eliminate unlawful discrimination;
- promote equality of opportunity;
- promote good relations between people of different racial groups.

There is also a specific duty to publish a Race Equality Scheme (RES); this should set out how a public body intends to meet the general duty and it must be reviewed every three years. Other specific duties include:

- assessing and consulting on the likely impact of proposed policies relating to the promotion of race equality;
- monitoring policies for any adverse impact relating to the promotion of race equality;
- publishing any results of any assessments, consultations and monitoring;
- ensuring public access to information and services are provided;
- training staff on the Race Equality Duty.

For the purposes of the Equality Act 2010 'race' includes colour, nationality and ethnic or national origins.

9.4.7 Religion or belief

Religious belief is a strong belief in a supernatural power or powers that control human destiny (Wikipedia)

Key legislation

- Equality in Employment Regulations (Religion or Belief) 2003
- Equality Act 2010

These regulations made it unlawful to discriminate on grounds of religion or belief, directly or indirectly, or to harass or victimise somebody because they have made a complaint or intend to, if they give or intend to give evidence to a complaint of discrimination. This applies to all aspects of employment (recruitment, term and conditions, promotions, transfers, terminations and training) and vocational training.

In relations to services, Part 2 of the Equality Act 2006 makes it unlawful for a public body involved in providing goods, facilities or services to discriminate on the grounds of religion or belief through:

- refusing to provide with goods, facilities or services if they would normally do so to the public, or to a section of the public to which the person belongs;
- providing goods, facilities or services of an inferior quality to those that would normally be provided, or in a less favourable manner or less favourable terms than would normally be the case.

The Equality Act 2010 includes any religion and it also includes a lack of religion. For example, an employee or jobseeker is protected if they do not follow certain religion or have no religion at all. Furthermore, a religion must have a clear structure and a belief system.

Belief means any religious or philosophical belief or lack of such belief. To be protected, a belief must satisfy various criteria, including that it is weighty and substantial aspect of human life and behaviour. Denominations or sects within a religion can be considered a protected religion or a religious belief.

Discrimination because of religion or belief can occur even where both the discriminator and recipient are of the same religion or belief.

9.4.8 Sexual orientation

Sexual orientation describes an enduring pattern of attraction – emotional, romantic, sexual, or some combination of these – to the opposite sex, the same sex, both, or neither, and the genders that accompany them. These attractions are generally subsumed under heterosexuality, homosexuality, bisexuality, and asexuality. (Wikipedia)

According to the American Psychological Association, sexual orientation also refers to a person's sense of 'personal and social identity based on those attractions, behaviors expressing them, and membership in a community of others who share them'.

Key legislation

- Equality in Employment Regulations (Sexual Orientation) 1975

These regulations made it unlawful to discriminate on the grounds of sexuality (gay or lesbian, heterosexual, bisexual), directly or indirectly, or to harass or victimise somebody because they have made a complaint or intend to, if they give or intend to give evidence to a complaint of discrimination. This applies to all aspects of employment (recruitment, term and conditions, promotions, transfers, terminations and training) and vocational training.

- Equality Act 2010

The Act protects bisexual, gay, heterosexual and lesbian people from acts of discrimination. In summary the Act sets out the different ways in which it is unlawful to treat someone, such as direct and indirect discrimination, harassment, victimisation and failing to make a reasonable adjustment for a disabled person. The Act prohibits unfair treatment in the workplace, when providing goods, facilities and services, when exercising public functions, in the disposal and management of premises, in education and by associations (such as private clubs).

9.4.9   Transgender

Transgender is a term used to describe people who may act, feel, think, or look different from the gender that they were born with. (Wikipedia)

Key legislation

- The Equality Act 2006
- The Equality Act 2010

The Gender Recognition Act 2004 gives transgendered or transsexual people full legal recognition of change of gender. It enables them to live fully and permanently in their chosen gender and to apply for legal recognition of that gender.

The Act allows for a transsexual person who has lived in their self-identified gender for at least two years, and who has a diagnosis of gender dysphoria (transsexualism), to obtain legal recognition of their gender for all purposes.

The Gender Equality Duty, of the Equality Act 2006 provides that transsexual people are explicitly covered in two elements:

- The first element of the duty, requiring public authorities to have due regard to the need to eliminate unlawful sex discrimination covers transsexual people, as unlawful sex discrimination includes the prohibition in the SDA on discrimination against transsexual people in employment and vocational training.
- The second element of the duty, dealing with promotion of equal opportunities between women and men, does not include specific obligation to promote equality of opportunity between transsexual people and people generally. However, transsexual people, as men or women, will benefit from the general obligation to promote equality of opportunity between the sexes.
- Legal protection for transsexual people was extended when the government implemented its commitment to bring in legislation to prevent discrimination against transsexual people in the provision of goods and services on 21 December 2007. The Discrimination Law

Review will be looking more broadly at the protection from discrimination for transsexual people.

The Equality Act 2010 provides protection for transgender people. A transgender person is someone who proposes to, starts or has completed a process to change his or her gender. The Act no longer requires a person to be under medical supervision to be protected – so a man who decides to live as a woman but does not undergo any medical procedures would be covered.

It is discrimination to treat transgender people less favourably for being absent from work because they propose to undergo, or are undergoing or have undergone gender reassignment than they would be treated if they were absent because they were sick or injured.

9.5   Anti-discriminatory practice

9.5.1   Promoting equality, diversity and rights

- When working with people with learning disabilities, it is essential that we consider the way in which we think about and treat them.
- Service users should be worked with in a way that demonstrates we accept them as individuals by respecting and valuing them and treating them equally.
- This is in recognition that service users have particular rights in the care they receive.
- Staff need to be aware of the rights of service users and be able to distinguish these from responsibilities.
- Staff would have to examine ways to ensure that service users have access to their rights.

This induction literature reflects on the meaning of rights, prejudice, stereotyping and discrimination and its effects.

9.6   Rights of service users

Rights can be divided into:

- *moral rights*: these are the rights that are not necessarily recognised in law, but are generally accepted as rights that we all have within our society; these include freedom of speech, of self-expression and freedom to protest;
- *sexual rights*: to express one's sexuality within the law;
- *employment rights*: to take meal breaks, have paid annual leave, have maternity leave and paternity leave;
- *citizens' rights*: to choose a GP, access personal information held about you, choose hospital treatment and to complain;
- human rights: generalised rights expressed in the Human Rights Act.

The rights of service users living in a care setting or their own home do not change; we include rights:

- to protection from abuse;

- to be independent;
- to be self-managing;
- to maintain status and self-esteem;
- to take calculated risks.

The exception to this is for service users who are sectioned under the Mental Health Act 1983 and therefore their right to liberty/freedom is restricted.

9.7   Legislation, policies, codes of practice and charters

These are used to uphold service users' rights. The rights of service users may come from the law, policies, codes of practice and charters. The purposes of these are:

- to guide the behaviour of people and organisations in ensuring rights of service users are upheld;
- whilst the law applies to everybody, different organisations will develop different policies for dealing with particular issues;
- to ensure an organisation works within what is considered good practice and current law.

(for example a health and safety policy will ensure that – if written accurately and followed correctly – both the employers and employees work within safe practice upholding the rights of staff and service users to a healthy and safe environment).

9.7.1   A care charter

A care charter is a document written by a care organisation setting out the standards a service user can expect from a service. It simply outlines the standards of care that the organisation provides, offers information about the health and social care services available and how to access them, and about how disagreements and grievances are settled. Whereas public charters, such as the Citizens' Charter outlines the rights that we should all be able to expect in our society.

9.7.2   Codes of practice

A code of practice refers to written guidelines which guide the practice of care workers, set by Skills for Care to help them comply with its ethical standards.

9.7.3   Legislations

The laws relating to rights and equality that are most relevant to care and those that you need to have a basic understanding of are summarised below.

- *Care Standards Act 2000*
  This sets out the minimum standards that care providers have to conform to and a range of rights that service users are entitled to.
- *Disability Discrimination Act 2005*
- *Equality Act 2010*

These set out the right not to be treated less favourably than able-bodied people in employment, access to education and transport, housing, goods and services.

- *NHS and Community Care Act 1990*
  Sets out the right of older and disabled people to have their needs assessed and services provided.
- *The Children's Act 1989*
  The Children's Act sets out the right to be protected from significant harm and also emphasises 'parental responsibilities' to the child rather than 'parental rights' over the child.
- *The Data Protection Legislation 1993*
  This protects the rights of all individuals to the privacy of information held about them.

9.8   Supporting service users in upholding their rights

You can help service users in upholding their rights by:

- listening – using your communication skills to accurately find out their needs;
- always ensuring that their needs are met promptly and in full;
- maintaining a pleasant attitude;
- ensuring that your communication is open and honest;
- developing a trusting relationship;
- ensuring you work within the service user's care plans;
- referring to legislation, codes of practice, policies and complaint systems to guide you in your practice;
- giving people information that they need – it is essential that this information is relevant, up to date and provided in a way that is appropriate to the service user – e.g. speech/vocalisation, signing, the use of Makaton, symbols/objects of reference for some service users with learning disabilities, TEACCH boards and translating information into community languages or large prints, taped or Braille forms of communication.

9.9   Constraints faced by service users

There will be occasions where service users are unable to fully exercise their rights. This may be for a range of reasons:

- physical barriers;
- disabilities and the particular nature of their learning disability;
- mental health status;
- emotional barriers such as lack of confidence;
- their rights being infringed by others;
- communication barriers.

9.10   Acting as an advocate (advocacy)

In some circumstances you may need to act as an advocate.

- This involves working closely with service users to find out their views and helping to represent them.
- It is important here that you communicate effectively to ensure it is their views you are accurately representing and not your own.
- On some occasion you may have to enable a service user to complain about the service.

9.11 Values and beliefs

- We are not born with values and beliefs but learn them through a variety of influences such as the culture we are brought up in, the views and attitudes of our parents, religion and the media.
- Our beliefs and values can be affected by our gender, age, abilities and disabilities, sexuality and religious beliefs or lack of them.
- Our values and beliefs are not fixed and are likely to change over time as we are subject to different experiences and influences.
- We share certain beliefs and values with others but we are all individuals with different experiences and therefore will have to develop our unique identity.
- We need therefore to ensure that we consider all service users as individuals and work with them accordingly.

It is the responsibility of a health and social care worker to ensure that they know the service users they work with and establish understanding of their individual identity, their values, beliefs and their preferences.

9.12 The meaning and effects of prejudice and discrimination

Prejudice usually comes out of knowing little about something or someone, but having strong ideas about it all the same. The word literally means pre-judging – jumping to conclusions. We are not born prejudiced but learn prejudices from an early age.

For example, if our parents are anti-gay then we may take those views on board. We are all likely to be prejudiced about something or other. However, as prejudice is learned it can also be unlearned by creating awareness – we are subject to other influences and have our own experiences as we develop and mature.

Discrimination is putting prejudice into action – where an individual is treated less favourably than others because of their social group to which they belong – this often occurs because of stereotyping.

Discrimination can occur both individually and institutionally:

- Acts of individual discrimination are often intended to have adverse impact on others because of their possession of certain traits.
- Institutional discrimination is built into the structure of the organisation itself. It can occur regardless of the desires or intentions of the people perpetuating it.
- To identify institutional discrimination we should not ask what the motives of the individuals involved are but what the results of their actions are.
- Institutional discrimination may be shown statistically. If a particular group is disproportionately absent in comparison to the pool of those possessing the relevant skills

or needs, discrimination is occurring even if it is impossible to document specific individual reasons.
- This can be seen in the context of:

  o your team at work;
  o overall workforce;
  o management levels;
  o the service users we support and serve.

9.12.1 Importance of recording and monitoring data

It is important to record and monitor data to remove discrimination in institutions.

- As institutional discrimination is built into the normal working relationships of our organisations, its continuation requires only that people continue 'business as usual'.
- Removal of institutional discrimination requires more than goodwill of assumptions and practices.
- Removal of institutional discrimination requires active review of the assumption and practices by which the organisation operates.
- Revision of those assumptions and practices may be found to have discriminatory results.

9.12.2 Kinds of discrimination

There are two kinds of discrimination;
- Direct discrimination
- Indirect discrimination

Direct discrimination

Direct discrimination is defined as treating a person less favourably than another based on disability, racial, gender, sexual orientation or religious grounds and includes segregation of a person on the above grounds.

Indirect discrimination

Indirect discrimination consists of applying, in the circumstances covered by the Act, a requirement or condition which although applied equally to persons of all racial groups, is such that a considerably smaller proportion of a particular racial group can comply with it than others, and it cannot be shown to be justifiable irrespective of the colour, race, nationality or ethnic or national origins of the person to whom it is applied.

Anybody can be discriminated against because of who they are or what they look like, or what their beliefs are, but certain groups in our society tends to suffer discrimination more often than others.

In order to reduce discrimination it is important to understand why it occurs.

9.12.3 Associative discrimination

Associative discrimination is discriminating against any individual or harassing them for their association with another individual who has protected characteristics. For example, if you look after someone who is elderly or disabled, you're already protected from being discriminated against, at work because of your association with the person you care for.

9.12.4 Perceptive discrimination

The Equality Act 2010 includes specific reference to perceptive discrimination against individuals for a perceived characteristic that they don't have. For example, if you tell your employer your husband's name is Mohammed, and your employer makes remarks to suggest that your husband is a terrorist, that would be perceptive race discrimination.

9.12.5 Why discrimination occurs

Discrimination occurs because of prejudicial assumptions that are based on lack of knowledge and understanding of those who are different from us.

- This can result in misconceptions about people.
- Embarrassment and misunderstanding about disability, sexuality, age and religion.
- Discrimination occurs because of fear and ignorance.

9.12.6 Why discrimination should be challenged

In accordance with the Health and Safety Executive (HSE) discrimination should always be challenged because many employers have found that making adaptations to their working practices to accommodate a diverse workforce makes good business sense.

It makes their business more attractive to both potential employees and customers and helps them recruit and retain the best people. This is not only good business sense but helps them meet the requirements of legislation.

Equally tackling discrimination in workplace is essential because:

- It is never acceptable whoever is involved.
- Because we are all human and prejudice is learned, it is likely that we are all prejudiced about something, because we have developed these attitudes from others, the media or personal negative experience.
- There will always be some groups with whom we feel more comfortable because we have some experience of them.
- It is essential that we reflect on these prejudices to try to overcome them so that they do not result in discriminatory actions against certain people we may be working with or supporting.

Some ways organisations may use to tackle discrimination
Some provisions that have helped in this respect include:

- extended leave for expectant mothers plus fraternal leave;
- religious holidays like Christmas, or Ramadan to mark end of fasting month of people of Islamic faith, or Diwali for Asian New Year celebrations;
- adaptation to hours of work: if an individual has a disability or long-term health condition, they may need to tell their employer so they can:
  o meet their health and safety responsibilities;
  o work with their employer on any 'reasonable adjustments' that may be needed, e.g. changing the working hours to include flexi-time, job-share, or starting and finishing later or earlier

9.12.7   Effects of stereotyping and discrimination

Stereotyping, labelling and discrimination can have very severe and lasting effects on people.

- Short-term effects can involve very negative feelings experienced by the person.
- Long-term effects include having access to services and facilities and participation in society restricted.
- If a service user with e.g. mental health problems is stereotyped and labelled mad, unstable and a danger to the society, others may also view this person in this way. The individual is likely to become isolated and take on board the label, believing themselves that they are mad, unstable and a danger to society.

Discrimination in care settings

- Lack of knowledge or misunderstandings about culture, religion or beliefs can lead to the needs of some service users not being met.
- Service users may have their rights withheld, especially the right to choose.
- There may be restrictions on access to and use of facilities and resources.
- Care workers may suffer discrimination from service users or colleagues.
- Access to training and learning may be restricted.

9.13   Disempowering and empowering care

9.13.1   Why is care sometimes disempowering?

There are a lot of reasons why care can be disempowering.

- On a personal level, care is sometimes given in terms of the carer's experience of care. Most people have experienced being cared for as children. Adults often take control and power over children because they assume that adults know best. If this is the carer's experience, it is so easy to slip into the role of disempowering.
- A carer assumes that anyone who gets care needs to be treated like a small child. The carer takes the power and the service user leaves all decisions to them.
- The service users may have their right to choice removed because disempowerment is what some carers have been used to doing.

- With disempowerment, there is danger that some carers might feel they need to have power over service users.
- Having control – not having to ask service users for their views can make the job simpler, quicker and easier.

9.13.2 What disempowerment does to people

1. When people believe they are being treated unfairly they become aggressive and may display challenging behaviour.
2. If people feel threatened that their lives are out of control, they usually feel frustrated and angry. If this anger is recognised and the situation is improved, the person may feel that they have been respected and that they can influence the situation. Very often this does not happen. Instead of recognising the service user's rights and needs, the service user's anger is seen as unreasonable or as a symptom of their illness.
3. Service users may withdraw into themselves while others may become aggressive and portray challenging behaviour.

9.13.3 Empowerment

Solomon (1976) provides a helpful definition when she writes of empowerment as:

> [a] process whereby persons who belong to a stigmatized social category throughout their lives can be assisted to develop and increase skills in the exercise of interpersonal influence and the performance of valued social roles. (p.12, cited in Dalrymple and Burke, 1995, p. 50)

9.13.4 Ways to empower service users

Empowerment for service users can be through use of occupational role and use of care plans. There are a number of ways you can empower a service user in your care:
1. Promoting anti-discriminatory practice by:
   - recognising stereotyping and assumptions;
   - educating service user about their rights;
   - understanding the local policies and guidelines;
   - understanding methods of challenging assumptions/discrimination.

2. Maintaining confidentiality:
   - understanding information systems;
   - identifying professional boundaries;
   - identifying decision making systems and support with decisions.

3. Supporting through effective communication:
   - understanding the effects of culture;
   - using active listening;
   - adopting a range of techniques to meet the service users needs, e.g. Makaton symbols, sign language, TEACCH, SPELL;
   - understanding constraints faced by service users.

4. Acknowledging individuals' personal beliefs and identity:
   - interpretation of power in role: you listen to people's beliefs and you support them in what their identity may be – for example, if they are homosexual or straight, or if they are religious or atheist, as a social care worker, you need to be able to listen to them and support them in their choice of belief;
   - identifying boundaries with own identity needs.

5. Promoting individuals' rights and choice:
   - through advocacy;
   - understanding legal and local perspectives;
   - understanding the principle of choice and boundaries;
   - understanding the factors which involve loss of rights.

9.14   Learning outcomes

- To understand what is meant by the term diversity
- To know the forms that discrimination and prejudice can take
- To understand the need to develop a work plan / action plan for improvement
- To know the reporting and feedback procedure

9.15   Framework for reflective practice

- ➢ *Knowledge:*   What have you learnt from reading this chapter?
- ➢ *Skills:*   What do you know, or can do differently now, that you did not/could not do before reading this chapter?
- ➢ *Practices:*   How can you perform a task now better than before?

9.16   References

Age UK: www.ageuk.org.uk

Bateman, N. (2000) *Advocacy Skills for Health and Social Care Professionals*. London: Jessica Kingsley.

Carers UK: www.carersuk.org

Citizens Advice Bureau. Website at: www.adviceguide.org.uk

Dalrymple, J. and Burke, B. (1995) *Anti-oppressive Practice: Social Care and the Law*. Milton Keynes and Philadelphia, PA: Open University Press, p. 50.

Daniels, L. and Macdonald, L.A.C. (2005) *Equality, Diversity and Discrimination: A Student Text*. London: CIPD.

Directgov: www.direct.gov.uk

Equality and Human Rights Commission: www.equalityhumanrights.com

Government Equalities Office website: www.equalities.gov.uk

Katherine A. (1993) *Boundaries: Where You End and I Begin: How to Recognize and Set Healthy Boundaries*. Seattle, WA: Parkside.

Kirton, G. and Greene, A.M. (2005) *The Dynamics of Managing Diversity. A Critical Approach*. 2nd edn. London: Elsevier-Butterworth-Heinemann.

Macdonald, L.A.C. (2004) *Managing Equality, Diversity and the Avoidance of Discrimination*. London: CIPD.

Solomon, B. Bryant (1976) *Black Empowerment: Social Work in Oppressed Communities*. New York: Columbia University Press.

Thompson, N. (2012) *Anti-discriminatory Practice: Equality, Diversity and Social Justice*. Practical Social Work Series. London: Palgrave Macmillan.

Thompson, N (2003) *Promoting Equality: Challenging Discrimination and Oppression*, 2nd edn. London: Palgrave Macmillan.

Thompson, N. and Thompson, S. (2008) *The Social Work Companion*. London: Palgrave Macmillan.

9.17   Induction workbook

1. Explain the meaning of the following terms? Give example of each.

    (a) Prejudice

    _____

    _____

    (b) Equal opportunities

    _____

    _____

2. It is important to support people in ways that respect their diversity because:

    _____

    _____

3. Explain three ways of enabling a service user to make informed decisions and choices.

    _____

    _____

4. What is likely to happen to a service user if you always make decisions on their behalf?

    _____

    _____

5. What kinds of difficulties do service users you work with, or will work with, face in their everyday lives, because of their disabilities?

    _____

    _____

6. How could society organise things differently to reduce or remove these difficulties for the people with disability?

    _____

    _____

7. Identify the laws which relate to protecting equality, diversity and rights of individuals (service users) when communicating with them.

    _____

    _____

8. Identify and explain how these laws are used in health and social care policies and procedures.

   _____

   _____

9. What is disempowerment and how does it come about in a care setting? How can you empower the service users you support?

   _____

   _____

PART III

THE EXPERIENCES AND PARTICULAR NEEDS OF SERVICE USER GROUPS

10 Types of Disabilities

AIMS

- To understand what learning disabilities are
- Types of disabilities physical (neurological disorders) mental illness
- To have an insight and support principles of each service user group
- To understand the nature of physical and mental illnesses and possible causes
- To understand how to support recovery in mental health

10.1 Learning disabilities

10.1.1 What is a learning disability?

A learning disability is a lifelong condition of intellectual disability often starting at an early age. It results in a reduced ability to learn new skills, understand complex information or live independently. Learning disabilities have a lasting effect on development socially and educationally, and can often be combined with physical conditions such as reduced functional skills.

The term 'service user groups' means similarities between the groups; these similarities are about the ways their disabilities are defined.

- Learning disability affects the way an individual learns, communicates or does some everyday things.
- A person with learning disability has this disability all through their life. There are many types of learning disabilities which can range from mild, moderate or severe.
- Some people with a mild learning disability do not need a lot of support in their lives. But other people may need support with all sorts of things, like getting dressed, going shopping, or filling out forms.
- Some people with learning disabilities also have physical disabilities. This can mean they need a lot of support 24 hours a day.
- A learning disability does not stop someone from learning and achieving in life, if they get the right support.
- There are many different causes of learning or profound and multiple learning disabilities. Often it is not possible to say why someone has a disability. But most are caused by the way the brain develops – before, during or soon after birth.

Before birth

- things that happen to the central nervous system (the brain and the spinal code, while a child is still in the womb);
- the mother having an accident or illness when she is pregnant;
- the genes that a parent passes on or how the genes develop while the unborn baby develops.

During birth

- when a baby does not get enough oxygen or born too early;
- when the baby experiences trauma during birth – baby delivered by ventouse (vacuum) or forceps.

After birth

- early childhood illnesses – meningitis;
- physical accidents;
- malnutrition;
- hereditary factors.

10.2 Autistic spectrum disorder (ASD)

The National Autistic Society (2010) definition is: 'Autism is a lifelong developmental disability. It is part of the Autism Spectrum and is sometimes referred to as Autism Spectrum Disorder or ASD.'

The word spectrum means a range of opinions, feelings etc. This term is used because no two people with autistic spectrum disorder are exactly alike.

- At one end of the spectrum are diagnostic terms such as 'Asperger's Syndrome', 'High Functioning Autism' and 'Pervasive Deficit Disorder'. At the other end of the spectrum there are terms such as 'Autism', 'Classic Autism' and 'Kanner Autism'.
- The term 'Autism Spectrum Disorder' is used because of the wide variation from person to person, depending on the severity and combination of each area of impairment.

Shore and Rastelli (2006) define autism as a neurological disorder caused by abnormalities in the brain. They further state that the autism spectrum is very broad and ranges from severe autism, where a child never learns to speak, to mild Asperger's syndrome, where a child has no obvious speech delay. The spectrum is continuous, ranging from a person who needs lifetime help with basic living skills to a college professor. They attribute the great variability to the extent of abnormalities in the brain.

In summary:

- Autistic spectrum disorder is a lifelong developmental disorder that affects the way a person communicates and relates to others. This may lead to difficulty in understanding that other people may see things from a different point of view.
- The person may have inflexibility in the application of rules that govern behaviour.
- The person may have repetitive enacting of role, often copied without understanding the purposes behind the action.
- The person may have difficulties in generalising concepts, which leads to inflexibility in the understanding of spoken language.
- The person may adopt routines and ritualistic behaviour which serve purposes to themselves and are acceptable so long as they do not cause harm to others.

Examples of repetitive routines are:

- pacing – a way to deal with stress and anxiety and to block out uncertainty;
- twiddling – a way to deal with sensory sensitivity;
- hand-flapping – may provide visual stimulation;
- finger-flicking;
- rocking – may be a way to stimulate the balance (vestibular) system;
- jumping – to offload sensory overload;
- spinning – a source of enjoyment and occupation;
- twirling;.
- repetitive questioning etc.

10.2.1   Tirade of impairment

People with autistic spectrum disorder have difficulties in three main areas within their lives: social imagination, social communication and social relationships; this is referred to as the Tirade of Impairment.

10.2.2   Impairment in imagination

Social imagination involves being able to predict other people's behaviour and imagine situations outside of a normal daily routine.

- People with autism have limited development of interpersonal play and imagination.
- They do not understand other people's point of view or feelings.
- They are agitated by changes in routine and often find change difficult and even upsetting.
- Any breaks in routine can cause immense anxiety or result in aggressive behaviour.
- They cannot generalise information.
- The limited range of imaginative activities may be pursued rigidly and often repetitively, e.g. repeatedly watching the same video/DVD.
- They have special interests, and may develop obsessive hobbies or collections, with support and encouragement these interests can be developed positively into areas of study or employment in their favourite subjects.
- They often prefer to order their day according to a set pattern, which provides continuity and stability to them.
- They take everything literally.
- People with Asperger's syndrome often excel at learning facts and figures, but find it hard to think in abstract ways.

10.2.3   Impairment in social relationships

Impairment in social relationships is a deficit in understanding how to behave and interact with other people and recognising the feelings of others and of themselves. Many people with Asperger's syndrome want to be sociable, but lack the social skills to interact in a conventional way. For example:

- inappropriate touching of other people;
- difficulty understanding and using nonverbal behaviour, e.g. eye contact, facial expressions and gestures;
- they may stand too close to people;
- they are unaware of the different ways to interact with friends, staff or strangers;
- people with autism have difficulties forming relationships; they often appear aloof and indifferent to other people;
- they may desire to have friends and relationships but struggle to initiate and maintain them.

10.2.4 Impairment in social communication

Social communication is the deficit in ability to communicate effectively with other people, which involves understanding and using verbal and nonverbal communication. People with ASD are unable to read facial expressions, gestures and social cues.

- They tend to ask repetitive questions.
- They cannot 'read between the lines' of what people mean.
- They talk about their own interests regardless of the listener's response.
- They make factual comments inappropriate to the context.
- They may lack the desire to communicate.
- They may communicate for their own needs, rather than for 'social' engagement.
- People with Asperger's syndrome may talk obsessively on a topic of interest to them and be unable to draw the conversation to an end independently.
- People with Asperger syndrome, despite often having good expressive verbal communication, may have difficulties in a two-way conversation; they may talk at you and have no interest in others' opinion if it doesn't coincide with their own.

10.2.5 Other traits displayed by a person with ASD

- They fixate on certain activities, word, songs or objects in an attempt to compensate or adapt to their inability to effectively connect meaning to others' words or actions.
- They cannot bear loud noises.
- They cannot bear to be touched.
- They experience mood disturbances, e.g. anxiety, aggression or depression.
- They may suffer from motor difficulties, e.g. walking on tiptoes, clumsiness.
- They experience attention difficulties, e.g. easily distractible.
- Sensory stimuli – people with autism may experience being over-sensitive (hypersensitivity) or under-sensitive (hyposensitivity) to any of the external or internal senses.
- People with hyposensitivity tend to seek sensation, where as those with hypersensitivity tend to avoid sensation.

10.2.6 Social blunders autistic people may unknowingly commit

- Blurting out embarrassing truths, for example 'your breath smells'.

- Talking about themselves without pausing to let other people talk.
- Taking things literally when a joke is being told.
- Delivering a one-sided monologue about their passion.

10.2.7 How to support people with autistic spectrum disorders

- Keep language clear and simple, and deliver in a calm manner.
- Avoid open-ended tasks or imaginative activities requiring abstract thoughts.
- Spell out clearly what you want an individual with ASD to do. Things that seems obvious to you do not to the individual with ASD. Their logic may be different to others.
- Maintain routines and rituals in the individual's support plans as these routines serve a purpose, and are acceptable as long as they do not cause harm to others.
- Ensure your approach with the service user is consistent at all times.
- Use positive instructions.
- Remove distractions and emphasise what is relevant.
- Use visual guides as appropriate e.g. activity timetable (avoid relying on the service user's memory).
- Establish the service user's area of interest.
- Maintain personal space and volume of speech.
- Build routines, ritualistic behaviour and special interests into learning.
- Re-teach social skills in each new setting as required. Repetition is the key to teaching new skills. Social skills include identifying proper behaviour, asking for assistance, maintaining topics, and reducing preservation (uncontrollably repeating a gesture, sound or phrase).

10.2.8 Elements of an autistic spectrum disorder friendly support task

- Use short tasks with frequent breaks.
- Keep rules and approaches consistent.
- Use appropriate language and rephrase written or verbal instructions as necessary. As individuals with ASD are very literal, don't presume that they can automatically read the insinuations in your language. Give clear specific instructions about what you want an individual to do.
- Always keep communication and messages simple. Avoid slang or jargon communication. A person who is autistic may find too much information hard to process within their immediate environment, which can lead to anxiety.
- Knowing the purposes of the task or activity and being able to see the outcome keep them engaged.
- Give sufficient time for instructions to be processed and understanding to be checked.
- Establish a rewards system; this could be available with the successful completion of the task.
- Use a lot of praise and encouragement each step of the way to motivate interest.
- Use visual reinforcement such as pictures, diagrams and demonstrations, e.g. TEACCH and SPELL devised by the National Autism Society and the University of Carolina

respectively. Individuals with ASD often wonder where to start; checklists and charts are a good starting point with timetables to give a structure of the day.

10.2.9 Social stories to support people with autistic spectrum disorders

Social stories were designed by Carol Gray (1994) to reinforce appropriate behaviour. They are short written stories to help the service user understand a small part of their social world and behave appropriately within it.

Social stories are vignettes designed to explain how social interactions work. They contain directives, descriptive, affirmative and perspective sentences.

- *Directive sentences* are used to suggest appropriate actions and instruct how to decode recognition. An example of a directive sentence: 'I will get on my pyjamas at 9.00 pm, so that I will be ready for bed at 10 pm.' The expected behaviour is to be in bed at 10 pm. The behaviour that will lead to the expected end is to have pyjamas on at 9.00 pm.
- *Affirmative sentences* are used to express commonly shared values or opinions of people in a given situation. An example of an affirmative sentence: 'It is good to listen to your key worker.'
- *Descriptive sentences* are logical and accurate, factual statements summarising the situation. An example of a descriptive sentence: 'We go for a gardening session every Thursday at 11.00 am.'
- *Perspective sentences* are used to describe the thoughts and feelings of other people. Occasionally perspective sentences may be used to describe or refer to the internal state of the person with an autistic spectrum disorder, e.g. 'The team leader is happy whenever I attend all my day's activities.'

10.2.10 Importance of social stories as a communication tool

- Each social story provides clear, concise and accurate information about what is happening in a specific social situation, outlining why it is happening and what a typical response might be in that social situation.
- Each social story aims to provide answers to key questions about a social situation that is problematic to the service user.
- An effective social story can enable a person to revisit the same social situation regularly, and remind them of their personal role in that social situation.
- Social stories are equally beneficial to staff because they learn to deal with, and alter the way they deal with, difficult social situations.
- They help staff develop more awareness that they are often a part of the problem, not just the answer.

The process of developing the story increases social understanding for both the person with autistic spectrum disorders and the person supporting those with autistic spectrum disorders.

10.2.11 Causes of challenging behaviour in children/adults with ASD

The first task is to understand, if possible, the reason for the challenging behaviour, rather than just focusing on the action. This is the key to achieving meaningful success in reducing the challenging behaviours. Most frequent reasons for challenging behaviour include:

- Communication – inability to understand explanations, instructions or information.
- Confusion and fear brought about by unfamiliar routines and situations.
- Lack of social skills – knowledge and understanding of the social rules of behaviour that govern social norms.
- Sensory impairment – oversensitivity to noise, bright lights, being touched, certain smells can be the cause of intense distress.
- Environmental factors – such as noise, heat, and cold or invasion of personal space – proximity of other people.
- Pressure to do tasks that are too difficult or go on too long or that are disliked.
- Inconsistency of support and response to challenging behaviour itself causes conflict and confusion
- Interference with the usual daily routine or individual's own repetitive routine without warning or prior warning.
- Although other reasons are more common, it is important to consider the possibility that challenging behaviour is due to discomfort, pain, illness, especially if it is different in form or timing from the usual pattern

10.2.12 Coping strategies for challenging behaviour

Coping strategies depend on the reasons for the challenging behaviour. They include:

- Structured, organised and predictable environment into the daily routine. An organised environment and routine are vital for individuals with ASD in order to give them a feeling of order and stability.
- The lack of ability to process information means that the person with ASD lives in a confusing and frightening unpredictable world. Staff should make sure they involve them by telling them very clearly what is going on, e.g. a visit to the GP, explain why they are waiting and what will happen next.
- Methods of communication have to be adapted to ensure that the individual understands what is required of them, e.g. use of alternative method of communication like sign language or communication aids like pictures, timetables etc. Keep checking things over to make sure they understand what is being communicated. This will minimise frustrations and prevent challenging behaviour.
- Ways should be sought to cope with aspects of the environment that causes distress (sensory impairment) such as noise levels, too bright lights.
- Avoiding pressure to perform tasks beyond the individual's abilities by breaking tasks into small manageable sizes and into easy steps to give the child/adult a sense of achievement.
- Maintaining good health care and watchfulness for signs of injury or illness like earache.

- Rewarding positive behaviour is more likely to be repeated while behaviour that is not rewarded is less likely to be repeated. However, if challenging behaviour cannot be prevented, it should not be rewarded.
- Timing is important. The response to behaviour, whether to be encouraged or discouraged, should be timed so that it is clear that it is that behaviour that produces the reward.
- Consistent approach in response to challenging behaviour should be maintained at all times to avoid confusion and re-enacting the behaviour.

10.2.13 Importance of understanding the cause of challenging behaviour

Understanding and making the connections between the challenging behaviours we observe and the causes of those behaviours helps create an insight that helps to develop ways of dealing with it, by using the A-B-C.

A   Antecedent is what happened just before the incident. Antecedents include learned patterns of behaviour, perceptions of cues or situations (self-talk), the immediate physical environment (temperature), air quality (heat/cold), food quality, the immediate social environment (peer interaction and behaviour), staff attitude, family interaction (visits, phone calls).

B   Behaviours – actions that follows the incident, head-banging, self-injurious behaviour, physical aggression and absconding.

C   Consequence – the outcome that follows a particular behaviour.

Keeping records and careful examination of the A-B-C patterns over a period of time can determine whether the consequence is affecting the particular behaviour with the desired results.

Using the A-B-C, staff can:

- predict – when it is known why behaviour occurs, staff can change the environment around the individual. changing behaviour to be most effective requires modifying antecedents, consequences, and thinking;
- plan – teach the individual new skills that they are lacking and alternative ways of behaving such as asking for assistance
- promote the positive behaviour and encourage its repetition;
- prevent the negative behaviour from happening;
- choose the most effective intervention strategies, by understanding the triggers of aggression.

10.2.14 Legislations and guidance supporting service users with ASD

- Disability and Equality Act 2010
- Autism Act October 2009
- Valuing Employment Now (VEN) June 2009 DoH – relates to no real jobs for people with learning disabilities
- White Paper: Building Britain's Recovery – relates to support for people with disabilities in training for and finding gainful employment
- Autism Education Act 2009

- Autism Strategy 'Fulfilling and Rewarding Lives'
- Human Rights Act (1998)
- Valuing People Now (2013)

10.3 Other types of disabilities

10.3.1 Mental (illnesses) health and legislation

People from all walks of life, at some stage in their lives will experience mental health problems. These can range from short-term periods of anxiety where they have insight into their feelings and behaviour to long-term severe illness which negatively affects every aspect of their lives.

For many people their experience of mental health problems will vary over the course of their lives and will therefore be mild or severe at different periods in time.

10.3.2 Mental Health Act (1983)

The Mental Health Act (MHA) makes it legal for people to be deprived of their liberty when they have neither committed a crime, nor appeared before a court of law. Once a person has been detained, they can be subjected to treatment which they would never have sought. MHA concerns:

- the admission of people to psychiatric hospitals against their will;
- their rights while detained;
- discharge from hospital and aftercare.

MHA, like any other law, is divided into sections, several of which are concerned with being compulsory admitted to hospital (hence the term 'sectioning').

10.3.3 Factors determining detention under Mental Health Act (1983)

People can only be detained if the strict criteria laid down in the Act are met which include:

- the person must be suffering from a mental disorder;
- people are detained because it is deemed to be in the interest of their own health and safety;
- because it is possible that other people may be at risk from the person's behaviour;
- when the person may have done themselves or anyone else any harm, or an informed suspicion;
- seen in a positive light, the Mental Health Act expresses society's concern and support for those with serious mental health difficulties;
- to protect the public from those acting apparently irrationally.

10.3.4 Sections of Mental Health Act (1983)

Section 1

- This section of the Mental Health Act explains what the Act is about and who it is intended to deal with.
- The Mental Health Act itself states that it deals with 'the reception, care and treatment of mentally disordered patients, the management of their property and other related matters'.

- Section 1 attempts to provide a legal rather than a medical definition of the types of mental health problems the Mental Health Act is intended to cover.
- Section 1 gives a definition of mental disorder, which is split into four types:
  - severe mental impairment
  - mental impairment
  - psychopathic disorder
  - mental illness

In broad terms, severe mental impairment and mental impairment relate to people with learning disabilities but only where this is associated with abnormally aggressive or seriously irresponsible conduct.

Psychopathic disorder is also clinically referred to as personality disorder.

For people with learning disabilities who are subjected to mental illness, the symptoms and experience can be compounded by autistic spectrum disorder (ASD).

Section 2

Section 2 of the Mental Health Act allows for the detention of a patient for up to 28 days for assessment, if this is thought appropriate by two doctors and approved by a social worker.

Section 3

Section 3 allows the detention of the patient for up to six months initially, but renewable for a further six-month period and then annually for assessment and treatment. However, the responsible medical officer (consultant psychiatrist) can discharge the patient from the section at any time during this period.

Section 17

- Allows a patient, who is currently liable to be detained in a hospital, to leave that hospital lawfully by being given leave of absence in accordance with the provision of Section 17.
- Only the patient's registered medical officer (RMO) with the approval of the Home Secretary in the case of restricted patients, can grant a detained patient leave of absence.

Documentation

When leave is granted, the following should be documented on Section 17 forms:

- the nature of the leave – escorted, unescorted, names of escorts;
- the number of escorts and gender of escorts if necessary;
- the level of observation whilst on Section 17 leave (i.e. in a group, 1:1 only or 2:1);
- whether the leave is one-off or regular (e.g. 4 hours every Wednesday to attend college);
- the period of leave;
- the locations to which the patient is allowed to travel (any restrictions on location or environment);
- the purpose of the leave (e.g. rehabilitation, leisure, treatment, education, employment, holiday, or home leave);
- the time and date of return;
- any other specific conditions.

Section 37

Section 37 is similar to Section 3 but is imposed by a court of law.

Sections 37/41

Features of Sections 37/41:

- imposed by court order with added restriction, with or without time limit;
- if time limited, it becomes unrestricted Section 37 at end of the period;
- with Sections 37/41, no renewals, but does need annual review;
- restrictions mean hospital cannot discharge, transfer or grant leave without the approval of the Home Office;
- medications may be given against patient's will if necessary.

Section 132 – Patients' rights

- Upon admission patients must be told why they are being detained, under which section and must be informed of their rights
- Information to include how to appeal against their section to the Managers Hearing and/or a Mental Health Review Tribunal
- Explain to the patient rights to complaints and procedure to Hospital Managers and to the Mental Health Act Commission
- Patient's understanding of the information must be checked and rechecked if necessary

10.3.5 Mental Health Capacity Act 2005

- This Act provides a framework to empower and protect vulnerable people who are not able to make their own decisions.
- The Act makes it clear who can make decisions, in which situation, and how they should go about this.
- It enables people to plan ahead for a time when they may lose capacity.
- The Act is underpinned by the following principles.
- Presumption of capacity – every adult has a right to make his or her own decisions and must be assumed to have capacity to do so unless it is proved otherwise.
- Individuals must retain the right to make what might be seen as eccentric or unwise decisions.
- The rights for individuals to be supported to make their own decisions – people must be given all appropriate help before anyone concludes that they cannot make their own decisions
- Least restrictive intervention – anything done for or on behalf of people without capacity should be the least restrictive of their basic rights and freedoms.
- Best interest – anything done for or on behalf of people without capacity must be in their best interests.

10.4   Mental health and mental illness

Mental health disorders are often classified in a medical context into two categories: psychosis and neurosis.

10.4.1 Psychosis

Psychosis is generally used to mean the presence of symptoms such as hearing voices. Anyone can have a short term period of psychosis due to, for example:

- bereavement;
- extreme stress; or
- a traumatic experience.

Causes

The cause of one-off episodes of psychosis may never be identified, but could be triggered by:

- drug use/misuse;
- biological conditions such as childbirth.

10.4.2 Neurosis

Neurosis is often used to mean an extreme version of a normal symptom such as extreme worrying. In the past it was used to mean that it was a lesser form of mental health problem but in fact severe depression can be as disabling as schizophrenia.

10.4.3 Schizophrenia

Schizophrenia is a severe mental disorder characterised by hallucinations, delusions, incoherence and physical agitation as defined in *The Diagnostic Statistical Manual of Mental Disorders* (1994) 4th Edition (DSM-IV).

- It is a 'thought' disorder.
- The first signs often appear when people are in their early twenties.
- The severity varies enormously but a large proportion of people affected will have intermittent, or continuous, symptoms throughout their life.
- Schizophrenia can affect people's thoughts, moods, behaviour and how they perceive the outside world.
- The risk people with schizophrenia face is killing themselves due to a range of factors including:

  o   side effects of medication;
  o   hearing voices;
  o   depression.
  o   lack of support.

10.4.4 Depression

Depression is a serious condition that involves the body, mood and thoughts (mind) according to DSM- IV.

- It affects the way a person eats, sleeps, the way they feel about themselves and the way they think about things.
- People with depression may not recognise that they have a treatable disorder or they may be discouraged from seeking treatment due to feelings of shame and associated stigma.
- Depression that is untreated or inadequately treated is associated with suicide.

There are three main types of depressive disorders:

- major depressive disorder;
- dysthymic disorder;
- bipolar disorder (manic-depressive illness).

Causes of depression

Depression can be a result of heredity but whether inherited or not depression is associated with:

- an imbalance in the brain chemicals;
- a combination of genetic make-up;
- psychological factors;
- environmental factors.

Factors involved in the onset of a depressive disorder

- Depression may also result from having a chronic physical illness.
- Use/misuse of certain medication or drugs.
- A relapse in people who have suffered previous depression; another episode may be precipitated by very little or no stress
- Stresses at work, at home or at school are other factors that may also trigger depression.

Symptoms of depression

DSM-IV gives the list of common symptoms as:

- severe low mood;
- lack of energy;
- poor appetite and sleep;
- poor concentration;
- feelings of hopelessness.

When depressed the person can experience feelings of guilt and that life is not worth living and have suicidal thoughts. The severity, duration and recurrence rate depends on treatment received, social situation and personality.

10.4.5 Bipolar disorder (manic depressive illness)

Owen and Saunders (2008) define bipolar disorder as a serious mental illness which is thought to be caused by an imbalance in the way the brain cells communicate with each other. This imbalance causes extreme mood swings that go beyond the normal 'ups and downs' of everyday life, wildly exaggerating the mood changes that everyone has.

Bipolar disorder involves severe mood swings which can significantly disrupt a person's life:

- Some people will persistently experience depression or mania and have very few episodes or none of the opposite state.
- The level of disability caused by this condition also varies; some people can have long or short periods of stability.
- Many people with this disorder hold down demanding jobs.
- A significant minority of people's lives are severely affected by it.

Symptoms of bipolar disorder (manic depression)

There's no 'typical' pattern of symptoms. It differs from person to person but according to DSM-IV, the typical symptoms include:

- fast speech and thinking;
- depression;
- delusions;
- extremely elated moods;
- over activity and disinhibition;
- self-harm .

Causes of bipolar disorder

Owen and Saunders (2008) include the following causes of bipolar disorder:

- Upbringing – such as traumatic childhood events.
- Misuse of drugs – such as cannabis. It has been known to trigger bipolar and other mental disorders.
- Stress – positive as well as negative events, for instance when stressed the body produces chemicals adrenaline 'fight or flight chemicals, but since the body does not need these chemicals to fight or run they remain in the body, and over time they damage health and well-being.
- Persistent lack of sleep can trigger bipolar disorder –According to one study 80% of psychiatric patients have sleep disorders, the severity of the insomnia matching up with the intensity of symptoms. Sleep is a powerful regulator of brain chemistry and people with bipolar commonly sleep too much, not enough, not at all or not deeply enough.
- In extremely rare cases, according to Professor Nick Craddock at Cardiff University, a head injury can be an external trigger of bipolar disorder: 'It depends on exactly what the injury is and what parts of the brain are involved, but head injury can bring on bipolar disorder in someone with genetic susceptibility. That's because head injuries can cause damage to some systems in the brain that are involved in the condition.'

10.4.6 Anxiety disorder

Anxiety is a universal human emotion but when it is severe and persistent it is regarded as an illness or disorder.

- Some people have generalised anxiety not related to specific events, but it is an unpleasant feeling that is with them all the time.
- Others experience episodes of anxiety which may have a specific trigger or occur spontaneously.

Symptoms of anxiety disorder

According to DSM-IV, the symptoms of anxiety disorder include:

- excessive worrying;
- paranoia;
- a racing heartbeat;
- feeling of dread and fear;
- sweating and shaking;
- repetitive tendencies such as an inability to leave the house without making endless safety checks on door locks.

10.4.7 Panic attacks

Panic attacks are associated with phobias and anxiety states, but they can occur spontaneously in people who have not previously experienced anxiety. They are characterised by:

- a sudden and intense sensation of fear;
- impending doom;
- frequently the person will feel they are going to die;
- the fear is accompanied by physical symptoms of:
  - breathlessness or hyperventilation;
  - tingling of the fingers;
  - tremor – trembling or shaking;
  - palpitations or a racing heart;
  - giddiness and sweating;
  - feeling unreal or detached from their surroundings.

10.4.8 Obsessive compulsive disorder (OCD)

Severe obsessive compulsive disorder is uncommon but people frequently complain of some features of the disorder. Some people have a combination of obsessional subjects and thoughts such as those about:

- personal safety;
- contamination;
- embarrassing subjects;
- compulsive behaviour.

Compulsions are:

- rituals;
- actions;
- mental processes that a person feels compelled to repeat to relieve anxiety and temporarily stop obsessional thoughts.

For example:

- a person may have an obsessional thought that their hands are dirty and repeatedly wash them over and over again.

10.4.9   Body dysmorphic disorder (BDD)

Body dysmorphic disorder (BDD) is defined by DSM-IV as a condition marked by excessive preoccupation with an imaginary or minor defect in a facial feature or localised part of the body. If a slight defect is present, which others hardly notice, then the concern is regarded as a markedly excessive. In order to receive a diagnosis, the preoccupation must

- cause significant distress;
- interfere in one's social or occupational life or ability to study.

10.4.10 Personality disorder

Personality disorder is a term applied to people who may have a range of difficulties coping with life and whose behaviour persistently causes distress to themselves and others.

- Personality disorders are associated with severe disturbances in the behavioural tendencies of an individual, usually involving several areas of the personality and always associated with social and personal disruption
- Personality disorders are inflexible and pervasive across many situations which the individual perceives to be appropriate.
- This behaviour can result in maladaptive coping skills, which may lead to personal problems that induce extreme anxiety, distress and depression.

There are different types of the disorders but common problems include:

- sustaining relationships;
- interpreting social clues.

Symptoms of personality disorder

1. *Suspicious*

- Paranoid; where the individual is suspicious of other people, sensitive to rejection and have a tendency to hold grudges.
- Schizotypal: this is where the individual has odd ideas and difficulties with thinking.
- Other people see the individual as eccentric.
- They may see or hear things.

2. *Emotional and impulsive*

- Antisocial: this is where the individual does not care about other people's feelings.
- They easily get frustrated and aggressive.
- May find it difficult to develop close relationships.
- May do things on the spur of the moment without feeling guilty.
- The individual may not be able to learn from their past unpleasant experiences.

3. *Borderline or emotionally unstable*

- This is where an individual does things without thinking.
- They find it hard to control their emotions.
- May feel empty inside or so bad about themselves that they resort to self-harming.
- They make relationships very quickly, but are unable to sustain them.
- The individual may feel paranoid or depressed and may even hear voices.

4. *Histrionic*

- This is where the individual tend to be self-centred and over-dramatise events.
- The individual has strong emotions, but quickly changes.
- They worry a lot about their appearances and crave excitement.

5. *Narcissistic*

- This is where the individual craves success, power and status.
- They seek attention positively or negatively.
- They exploit others for their own gain.

6. *Anxious*

- Obsessive-compulsive: this is where the individual is a perfectionist.
- They worry about the details in everything.
- They are cautious and find it hard to make decisions.
- They have high moral standards,
- They worry about doing the wrong thing and judge other people.
- They are insensitive to criticism.
- They may have obsessional thoughts and behaviour.

7. *Dependent*

- This is where an individual relies on other people to make decisions for them,
- They do what other people want them to do.
- They find it hard to cope with daily tasks,
- They may feel hopeless and incompetent.
- May easily feel abandoned by others.

10.5   How to support recovery for people with mental illnesses

Whereas specialist healthcare professionals provide diagnosis and treatment, social care workers through awareness and understanding (training) provide hope and empowerment through effective services and support with the guidance of a multidisciplinary team (MDT) who formulate the development of support plans for the service users identifying what types of support may be useful. The aim of these guidelines is to empower social care workers working in mental health services, and to focus on the well-being of the service users within a care environment.

10.5.1   What is recovery?

Recovery is classified into two categories; clinical and personal recovery.

Clinical recovery

Clinical recovery is an understanding that has emerged from professional-led research and practice, and involves 'getting back to normal' – being symptom-free, in employment or education, living independently, having friends, *etc.* (South London and Maudsley NHS Foundation Trust),

Personal recovery

Personal recovery is an idea that has emerged from the expertise of people with lived experience of mental illness, and means something different to clinical recovery. The most widely used definition of personal recovery is from Anthony (1993):

> a deeply personal, unique process of changing one's attitudes, values, feelings, goals, skills, and/or roles. It is a way of living a satisfying, hopeful, and contributing life even within the limitations caused by illness. Recovery involves the development of new meaning and purpose in one's life as one grows beyond the catastrophic effects of mental illness.

10.5.2   The possibility of successful recovery

Promoting hope

One of the key factors in successful recovery from any illness is hope – the belief that things can get better, given time. Staff should support individuals to generate feelings of hope or the possibility that they will be able to successfully recover.

The probability of success goes up any time people choose attitudes and actions that are both within their control and also increases the likelihood of getting what they want either now or in future. Things like displaying stories of recovery, supporting people to re-engage in determining their own future, distributing information written for service users about recovery and inviting peer support specialists (who provides visible role models of recovery) to participate in service users goals and dreams. This not only makes their chances of success of recovery more likely in reality, but they make it more believable in their minds and hearts, increasing their will to recover by making the path to success more and more apparent.

10.5.3 A sense of control

The feeling of being in control, of having a say in what happens in one's life, has far-reaching consequences for the physical and mental health and well-being of people. Increasing the sense of control among service users in hospitals, rehabilitation and treatment centres, or those living in supported accommodation, will make them feel valued, confident, comfortable and able to make decisions for themselves. The increased control can be from simple changes, such as the physical environment; organisational culture, the attitudes and behaviour of staff, allowing the service user to decide what they would have for meals, among other things.

By taking control over even the simplest elements of the individual's environment or treatment, access to therapy, talking with the individual about their life, what they want from admission, what they hope to do after, increases the likelihood of the individual experiencing well-being in their everyday lives.

10.5.4 Focusing on past success

The perception of one's ability increases when we start to focus on what we do that's working, and along with it we increase the possibility of success. It is the same for recovery.

10.5.5 Lowering sights (expectations)

While conventional wisdom tells us to shoot for the stars, successful recovery research points out that lowering our sights and focusing on a target that we know we can achieve can quickly turn even the most daunting challenge into a fun adventure. As a person's confidence and skills increase, the target can gradually turn to the original expectations. For many people with mental illness, they need support to understand that recovery involves innumerable small acts and that it happens in stages.

10.5.6 Clear goals

Having a clear goal, purpose or intention acts as a sort of organising principle for our attention, filtering our experience down from a world of infinite possibilities to a selective collection of experiences which allow us to focus, feel in control, 'make sense' of what is happening to us and respond deliberately. Therefore, the simplest way to transform any task into positive potential experience is to support people's set intention, purpose or goal in relation to that task.

- Staff should primarily focus on identifying, elaborating and supporting work towards the person's goals. If people are to be responsible for their own lives, it means avoiding the imposition of meanings and assumptions about what matters, and instead focussing on the person's life goals.
- Goals, purposes or intentions are strengths-based and oriented towards reinforcing a positive identity and developing valued social roles.
- Staff can support the use of user-developed workbooks – Wellness Recovery Action Planning (WRAP). WRAP® was developed by a group of people who have a lived experience of mental health difficulties; people who were searching for ways to resolve issues that had been troubling them for a long time. WRAP® involves listing your personal resources, your wellness tools, and then using those resources to develop action plans to use in specific situations which are determined by you. WRAP® is adaptable to

any situation and includes a crisis plan or advance directive. For more details see www.mentalhealthrecovery.com

10.5.7   Promoting and encouraging physical activities

An active lifestyle is key to improving and maintaining health. Physical activities reduce risks of chronic diseases and can benefit mental health by reducing feelings of depression and anxiety. People with mental health disorders are likely to face particular barriers achieving an active lifestyle. This can relate to lack of health education and awareness, lack of confidence and difficulties in accessing sports facilities.

Staff can help service users to overcome these barriers by filling gaps in their learning and creating opportunities for them to participate in physical activities. The best way to capture someone's interest in physical activity is to ask them what they would want and encourage them to take ownership. This could include:

- inviting a qualified aerobics, yoga or dancing teacher to run a session within the hospital/project;
- staff making links with local authority leisure centres to obtain free or subsidised access to swimming pools, gyms and other leisure facilities;
- working with charitable organisations to enable people to attend an outdoor activity centre and try their hands in gardening, pottery etc.;
- making links with local professional sports teams – people can gain inspiration and motivation from watching and interacting with professional players.

10.5.8   Promoting healthy eating

Enabling people to access and maintain a balanced diet can bring huge benefits to their physical, mental and emotional health. People should have choices about what they eat and be involved in planning and designing menus as much as possible. It is also important that food is presented and served in a way that makes people feel valued. Friendly staff and quality crockery can go a long way in creating a homely and nurturing environment for patients/service users in a hospital/rehabilitation projects/supported housing.

10.5.9   Promoting mental and emotional well-being

Due to negative experiences and stigma associated with mental health disorders, many people suffer before getting help; by then they have reached crisis point. There are many ways that staff can positively promote the mental and emotional health of service users. This can entail the following:

- Group and one-to-one work to raise people's awareness and understanding of mental (illness) health – including work to tackle the stigma surrounding mental illness and to help them recognise the signs of mental health problems.
- Mental health professionals should aim to reduce stigma surrounding mental illness by using language people can understand to encourage them to recognise and deal with issues on which they may be holding back.
- Peer-support schemes that empower people to provide support and advice to others going through a common experience.

- Work to build people's emotional resilience and coping skills – this might include sessions on stress management, self-defence, assertiveness and anger management.
- Enabling people to access professional counselling by making links with external counsellors or supporting existing staff to become trained counsellors.
- Promoting self-help websites and telephone help lines such as Saneline.
- Encouraging people to attend activities organised by support peers groups such as gardening as this can have therapeutic effect.
- Organising regular trips to theatres, cinema, parks and places of interest to stimulate people's curiosity and prevent boredom.
- Relaxation sessions incorporating hair, and beauty and alternative therapies such as yoga, reflexology and massage.
- Groups and individuals to work to prevent and respond to bullying and violent behaviour, such as interventions to support victims gain confidence and assertiveness skills.
- Developing joint working protocols and service-level agreements can help ensure people experiencing mental health problems receive the support they need. Details of local services can be obtained from local mental health trust – GPs who can provide and coordinate support via primary care and community services to people such as those suffering bereavement, stress or anxiety.
- Creating an environment that promotes people's self-esteem, confidence and motivation should help prevent underlying mental health problems from escalating, and empower people to feel in control of their lives and future choices. The overall atmosphere within a project/rehabilitation centre has a big impact on how people feel. People feel happy and more secure when they know that staff are accessible and have time to listen to them
- Immediate feed: Tailoring practice through performance feedback. Without good information about success, the natural tendency is to assume all is well. People thrive on having clear goals and making constant adjustment in pursuit of that goal. Giving continual feedback is a way to check whether the person is on track.

10.5.10 Diversity and inclusion

The physical environment is important and should be inclusive of all people; staff should work with service users to promote their health and well-being, and recognise their diverse needs.

Information should be made available in a range of formats so it is accessible and sufficiently visual for people who do not speak English well or have poor literacy skills. Similarly, activities should be pitched at a level that enables people of all abilities to participate fully. The cultural appropriateness of health messages and interventions also need to be carefully considered.

10.5.11 Building positive relationships

Positive relationships that are based on mutual trust and respect are essential foundations for work to assess and address people's need to feel valued and safe, to be able to talk openly about their needs and to feel confident about seeking and receiving help.

Staff should encourage and promote peer relationships. This can be to inform of peer support specialists, mutual self-help groups like Restore and peer-run programmes, which all have one goal in common: they directly communicate the message that the experience of mental illness is an asset, and their central goal is to support people to re-engage in determining their own future.

Relationships with professionals

Mental health professional should aim to reduce stigma surrounding mental illness by using language people can understand to encourage them to recognise and deal with issues on which they may be holding back. Professional expertise support self-management in which the processes of assessment, goal-planning and treatment all support recovery.

10.5.12 Promoting mental and emotional health

There are two main aspects of work to promote positive mental and emotional health. First is to work to identify and meet the needs of people whose behaviour suggests underlying diagnosable mental health problems.

The second is creating an environment that promotes people's self-esteem, confidence and motivation. Staff should have understanding of mental health problems and be equipped to identify a person may be unwell and in need of further support from mental health services. Without this knowledge, problems may not be detected until a person reaches a crisis point.

People may be reluctant to seek help or talk about their mental and emotional health from fear and misconceptions about mental illness. To challenge this, it is important that staff talk to people about their mental health in a way and style that is nonthreatening, and to develop activities that include and address mental health issues.

Good links between supported housing projects, floating mental health workers and local specialists mental health teams should help to ensure people have easy access to specialists mental health teams for instance community mental health teams (CMHTs), especially those who experience more serious problems including depression, bipolar disorders, schizophrenia, eating disorders and self harm.

Staff should work together to agree how individual people would be supported and, where necessary, develop joint care plans. Some supported housing projects have built capacity to address people with mental health needs by employing specialists' mental health workers, alongside generic staff, or arranging for mental health nurses to practice regular outreach services.

Other housing projects where people with mental health problems are housed have identified a project worker/mental health rehabilitation officer to lead on mental health promotion with remit for developing proactive links with services, coordinating resources and organising mental health training and awareness.

These different approaches all have the same aim of ensuring that people have quick access to specialist assessment that are linked in with additional services as needed, and that staff are supported to gain confidence and skills to meet people's mental health needs and support recovery.

10.6   Neurological disorders

Neurological disorder is a disorder of the body's nervous system, structural, biochemical or electrical abnormalities in the brain, spinal cord or in the nerves leading to or from them. (http://www//dixiex.com). Neurological disorders include:

- disorders involving muscles;

- structural disorders of the brain and spinal cord;
- structural disorders of the nerves in the face, trunk and limbs;
- conditions which are not caused by structural disease such as many varieties of headache;
- conditions such as epilepsy, fainting and dizziness which are often caused by disordered physiology, rather than abnormal anatomy.

Neurological disorders affect people's ability to think and control their actions, and are particularly distressing, both for the patients, their families and carers.

10.7 Epilepsy

Epilepsy is a neurological disorder marked by sudden recurrent episodes of sensory disturbance, loss of consciousness, or convulsions, associated with unusual electrical activity in the brain (www.epilepsysociety.org.uk). Epilepsy is a physical condition that starts in the brain.

- When the workings of the brain are disrupted a person may suddenly have a seizure.
- Many people will have a single seizure at some time in their lives, but this does not mean that they have epilepsy.
- If a person has epilepsy it means they have had more than one seizure that began in the brain.
- Some people call their seizures by different names – such as a fit, funny turn, attack, or blackout.
- An epilepsy seizure happens when ordinary brain activity is suddenly disrupted.

Epileptic seizures can take many forms, since the brain is responsible for such a wide range of functions, including:

- personality;
- mood;
- memory;
- sensations
- movement and consciousness.

Any of these functions may be temporarily disturbed during the course of a seizure.

10.7.1 Scope of epilepsy

There are many different types of seizures:

- Not all of them involve convulsions.
- A person with epilepsy can experience more than one type of seizure.
- The frequency, length and pattern of seizures tend to be fairly constant for each individual, although it may change in the longer term.
- If a person becomes aware of any changes to their seizures it may be helpful to have a review of their epilepsy and its treatment.
- Anyone can have epilepsy; it occurs in all ages, ethnic backgrounds and social classes.

10.7.2   Causes of epileptic seizures

The reasons why some people develop epilepsy are not straightforward and there are many possible causes which can include:

- head injury;
- infections of the brain such as meningitis;
- a stroke;
- brain damage caused by a difficult birth;
- a scar on the brain; images from scans of the brain may show what the cause is.

10.7.3   Types of epilepsy

There are two types of epilepsy, one with known cause and the other unknown.

- 'Idiopathic' epilepsy is epilepsy where there is no known cause
- 'Symptomatic' epilepsy is epilepsy with a known cause, these include:
  o   brain damage caused by a difficult birth;
  o   brain injury during an accident;
  o   a severe blow to the head;
  o   a stroke;
  o   an infection of the brain such as meningitis;
  o   very occasionally a brain tumour.

10.7.4   Treatment

The response to drug treatment can vary from person to person.

- Up to 70% of people with epilepsy could have their epilepsy controlled with anti-epileptic drugs (AEDs).
- Anti-epileptic drugs (AEDs) prevent seizures from happening, but do not cure epilepsy.
- There are many anti-epileptic drugs (AEDs), and the type someone takes will depend on the type of seizures they are having.

10.7.5   Types of epileptic seizures

Epileptic seizures can be divided into two main types:

- partial seizures;
- generalised seizures.

Seizures can vary from one person to another and how people are affected and recover varies after seizures.

10.7.6   Partial seizures

- In partial seizures the seizure starts in, and affects, just part of one side of the brain.
- In a partial seizure what happens during the seizure depends on where in the brain the seizure happens and what this part of the brain normally does.

10.7.7 Simple partial seizure (SPS)

In a simple partial seizure:

- the person is conscious (awake) and aware of what is happening to them;
- there could be twitching of one limb or part of a limb;
- there could be an unusual smell or taste in the mouth;
- there could be a strange feeling such as a 'rising' sensation in the stomach or 'pins and needles' in the part of the body;
- there could be a sudden intense feeling of fear or joy;
- the person could have problems speaking or understanding;
- the person could experience sexual feelings and show sexual behaviour;
- screaming, swearing or crying out;
- losing control of their bladder and/or bowels.

What to do during seizure

Although the person is awake and aware, simple partial seizures can feel unsettling so:

- giving gentle reassurance may be helpful.

10.7.8 Complex partial seizures (CPS)

A complex partial seizure (CPS) affects a bigger part of the brain than a simple partial seizure and may last from a few seconds to a few minutes. In a complex partial seizure:

- the person's consciousness is affected and they may be confused;
- they might wander around;
- they may behave strangely like fiddling with their clothes;
- they may not know what they are doing;
- they may pick objects up for no reason;
- they may make chewing movements with their mouth;
- afterwards, they may need to sleep;
- they may be confused/disoriented for some time;

What to do during the seizure

- Do not restrain the person as this may upset or confuse them.
- Gently guide them away from any danger (such as walking into the road).
- Speak quietly and calmly so that they are not startled.
- They may be confused; therefore if you speak loudly or act forcefully this may confuse them more.
- They may mistake your help for being hostile.
- They may be upset or respond in an aggressive way.
- If you don't know what to do or are not epilepsy trained or have no epilepsy awareness call the paramedics – dial 999.

After the seizure stops

- the person may feel tired and need to sleep;
- it may help if you remind them where they are because they may be confused and disoriented and may not be fully aware of their surroundings;
- stay with them until they have recovered, and can safely return to what they were doing before the seizure;
- some people recover quickly after their seizure while others may take longer to feel back to normal again.

10.7.9 Secondarily generalised seizures

- A secondarily generalised seizure starts as a partial seizure and then becomes a generalised seizure.
- Some people call their partial seizures an 'aura' or 'warning' because it warns them that a generalised seizure may follow.
- When this happens the person becomes unconscious and will usually have a tonic clonic seizure.

What to do during the seizure

If the person is aware of a warning, they may need help to make themselves safe before the generalised seizure starts, e.g. lying on the bed or staying at home.

10.7.10 Generalised seizures

Generalised seizures affect both sides of the brain:

- the person becomes unconscious;
- afterwards the person will not remember what happened during the seizure.

The main types of generalised seizure are absence, atonic, myoclonic, and tonic-clonic seizures.

10.7.11 Absence seizures (sometimes called petit mal)

During an absence seizure a person:

- becomes unconscious for a short amount of time, usually a few seconds;
- they may look blank and not respond to what is happening around them; for example, if they are walking they may continue to walk, but will not be aware of what they are doing.

What to do during the seizure

- Stay with the person.
- Gently guide them away from any danger.

10.7.12 Atonic seizures (sometimes called drop attack)

In an atonic seizure:

- the person's muscles suddenly become stiff;
- if they are standing they often fall backwards/forward and may injure the back of their head or their face;
- the person's muscles suddenly relax, and they become floppy;
- the seizure tends to be very brief and happen without warning so you cannot help during the seizure itself'
- people usually recover quickly.

What to do after the seizure

- As the person recovers they may need reassurance.
- If they have been injured, they may need medical help.

10.7.13 Myoclonic seizures

- Myoclonic seizures involve the jerking of a limb or part of a limb.
- They often happen shortly after waking up from sleep.
- They are brief and can happen in clusters with many happening close together in time.
- As they are so brief, there is nothing that needs to be done to help the person other than making sure they haven't hurt themselves.

10.7.14 Tonic clonic (convulsive) seizures (sometimes called grand mal seizures)

- During a tonic clonic seizure the person goes stiff, usually falls to the ground shakes or makes jerking movements (convulses).
- Their breathing can be affected and they may go pale or blue, particularly around their mouth.
- They may also bite their tongue.
- Some people have just clonic (convulsive) seizures.

Although a tonic clonic seizure can be frightening to see, these seizures are not usually a medical emergency. Usually, once the jerking has stopped, the person recovers and their breathing goes back to normal.

What to do during the seizure

- *Try* to stay calm.
- Check the time to see how long the seizure is going on for (because there may be a risk of *status epilepticus* – see notes below).
- Move objects, such as furniture away from the person in case they hurt themselves.
- Only move them if they are in a dangerous place; for example, at the top of stairs or in the road.
- Put something soft (like a jumper/pillow) under their head, or cup their head in your hands, to stop it hitting the ground.

- Do not restrain them, allow the seizure to happen.
- Do not put anything in their mouth – there is no danger of them swallowing their tongue during the seizure (this has been medically proven).
- Try to stop other people from crowding around if you are in a public place.

What to do after the seizure stops

When the jerking (convulsing) has stopped:

- Roll them on to their side into the recovery position (see next section on how to put someone in a recovery position).
- Wipe away any spit and if their breathing is difficult, check their mouth to see that nothing is blocking their airway, like food or vomit.
- Try to minimise any embarrassment. If they have wet themselves, deal with this as privately as possible; put a jacket or blanket over them.
- Stay with them, giving reassurance, until they have fully recovered.
- Some people recover quickly after these seizures but more often the person will be very tired and may want to sleep.
- Some people may not feel 'back to normal' for several hours or sometimes days.

10.7.15 How to put someone into the recovery position

Barraclough (2012) advises the following:

When an unconscious person is lying on their back, there are two main dangers that can compromise (block) the airway:

- the tongue: tongue touching the back of the throat;
- vomit: if the person is sick.

By placing the person in the recovery position, the tongue will not fall backwards, so it won't block the airway. If the person is sick (vomiting), the vomit will run out of the corner of the mouth and keep the airway clear.
- Kneel beside the person (service user) and make sure that both their legs are straight.
- Place their arm nearest to you at right angles to their body, elbow bent with the palm facing upwards.
- Lift their other arm across their body putting the back of their hand against their cheek nearest you. Hold it there with your hand.
- Using your other hand, lift the knee furthest from you, and pull it upwards so that their leg is bent and their foot is flat on the floor.
- Keeping their hand against their cheek, pull the bent knee towards you. This will roll them onto their side.
- Keep the knee bent and position this leg at a right angle to their body.
- Make sure their airway is open: gently tilt their head back and lifting their chin check that nothing is blocking their throat and that they are breathing.
- Call for an ambulance if this has not already been done.
- Check breathing regularly. If the breathing stops before the ambulance arrives, turn the patient onto his back again, and perform resuscitation (CPR).

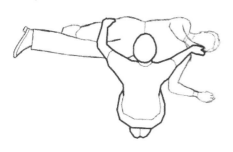

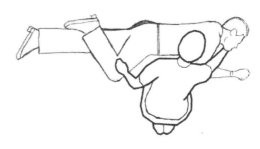

1. Keep the person's hand pressed against their cheek and pull on the upper leg to roll them towards you and onto their side.

2. Tilt the head back so they can breathe easily.

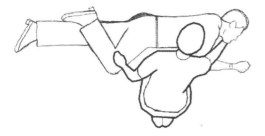

3. Make sure that both the hip and the knee of the upper leg are bent at right angles.

Figure 10.1 How to put someone into the recover position.

Healthy tips

- If the victim is pregnant, be sure to put her on her left side. Otherwise, her uterus might apply pressure on major arteries, possibly leading to death.
- If the victim has wounds on the torso, position them on the side that puts the wounds closer to the ground. This reduces the likelihood of blood affecting both lungs (wikiHow)

10.7.16 *Status epilepticus*

- Most people's seizures last the same length of time each time they happen, and usually stop by themselves. However, sometimes seizures do not stop, or one seizure follows another without the person recovering in between.
- When a seizure goes on for 30 minutes or more, it is called *status epilepticus*, or 'status' for short.
- Status can occur in any type of seizure and the person may need to see a doctor. However, *status epilepticus* in a tonic clonic (convulsive) seizure is a medical emergency.
- It is important to call for an ambulance before the seizure goes on too long.
- Do not wait until it has lasted 30 minutes before calling for help.
- Some people who go into status are prescribed emergency medication, either rectal diazepam or Buccal Midazolam, to stop their seizures.

As a carer you need to be trained on how to give emergency medication and it is important to have a written protocol (care plan) for each individual, for you to follow.

How else can you help?

- Checking the length of a seizure is essential in avoiding *status epilepticus.*
- Another important reason to check the time and note the length of a seizure is so that you can pass this information on afterwards to the person's doctors or paramedics.
- Many people keep a record of their seizures, and a description of the seizure and how long it lasted.
- The recorded information is vital for them to pass on to their specialist which is useful for treatment and medication review.

10.7.17 Safety guidelines for individuals with epilepsy

Safety is important for everyone. Most people with epilepsy can be supported to live a full and active life by thinking about extra safety measures. These extra safety measures depend on the types of seizures the person has and their living arrangements. (Epilepsy Society, 2011)

Inside the home

Making the home or living space safer may lower the number of accidents that could result from a fall during a fit.

In the lounge

- Furniture; when choosing furniture it's essential to think about how they might hurt the service user if they fall against them during a seizure.
- Flooring like ceramic tiles could cause serious injuries if a service user was to fall against them.
- Coarse fabrics could cause burns, therefore it is important for soft fabrics.

Soft furnishing

- In areas where food may be spilt, non-slip rugs, carpets, and tiles should be fitted.
- Fabrics that are easy to clean would be useful.
- Fire-resistant fabrics and furniture should be used more commonly, especially if the individual smokes.
- Fitting protective covers over corners on furniture reduces injury of cuts, bruises and broken bones if the individual falls on the furniture.
- Fitting radiators guards reduces injury if the individual falls against them and receives burns from them when hot.
- Buying round tables may help to reduce injury if the individual falls against them and buying coffee tables fitted with shatter-proof fibre glass to prevent shattered glass from cutting the individual were they to fall on it.

Glass

- Safety glass in doors and low windows is now a legal requirement in new buildings which can greatly reduce the risk of injury if a service user falls against them.

- Replacing old glass with safety glass (shatter proof) in old homes may greatly reduce the risk of injury should the individual fall against them.
- Fitting old glass with safety glass film which stops the glass from splintering when it is broken should the individual falls against them.

Smoke detector

- Having a smoke detector and testing it regularly is important for the service users and everyone.
- Having a seizure while smoking could result in a fire and a smoke detector will raise the alarm and save the individual.

Heating the home

Heating the home should be undertaken and a risk assessment carried out. The following tips may lower the risk of injury if someone has a seizure:

- Central heating of the home with heat sensors to regulate the heating to a standard requirement.
- Cover hot pipes with lagging to help prevent burns/injury if they are gripped or fallen against.
- Radiator guards can help stop the individual falling on to or gripping the radiator.
- Using heaters that are secured to the wall or floor so that they cannot be knocked over.
- Using fire guards that can be secured to the floor in front of an open fire to help prevent the individual from falling into the fireplace.

In the kitchen

For safety in the kitchen the following measures can reduce injury:

- To avoid knocking pans and pots from the cooker, turn the saucepan handles to the side.
- Use the back burners rather than those at the front of the cooker.
- Grill food rather than fry it.
- Where possible use a hob on which the heat can be turned off quickly, such as gas or halogen hob.

To reduce the risk of scalds and burns

- Encourage the service user to limit carrying hot food to short distances
- Use a trolley to move food and hot dishes from the oven to tables instead of carrying them.
- Use a cordless kettle with a hinged lid that 'locks' into position and which switches itself off automatically when it reaches a boiling point.
- Use a safety cradle that allows the kettle to be tipped gently so hot water can be poured without the need for lifting the kettle.
- Use low-level grill instead of eye-level grills. An eye-level grill could increase the risk of injury to the face if the individual had a seizure while using it.

- Fitting a cooker guard around the front of the hob so that heat sources are harder to touch by accident.
- Using a tumble dryer may reduce the need for ironing clothes by using anti-creasing to reduce creases.

Microwaves

Microwaves are safer than other ovens when they are cooking or heating up food because:

- Microwaves don't get warm to touch, which means they are unlikely to burn someone if they touched while having a seizure.
- They automatically switch off when the time is up. This means that if the microwave is left unattended there is less chance of food burning or a fire starting.
- To avoid the likelihood of people burning themselves when taking hot food out of the microwave, it is important to use microwave-proof containers to cook or reheat food.
- Microwaves can be used to heat mugs of water for hot drinks instead of using a kettle.

In the bathroom

Great care needs to be taken when bathing people with epilepsy to minimise injuries.

- Having a shower is safer than having a bath because the water drains away and this lowers the chances of the person drowning if they had a seizure while getting washed.
- A fitted seat designed for use in the shower can stop a person from falling during a seizure.
- Soap trays should be set into the wall instead of sticking out, which can reduce the injuries if a fall happens.
- Shower curtains might be easier to remove and get a person out if they need to be moved, unlike high-sided bases as water can be trapped if the drain is covered.

In the bath

In the event that the individual who has seizures chooses to have a bath or there is no alternative, the following measures can help reduce risks:

- Run a shallow bath and put cold water in before the hot water to help prevent burns if a seizure happens.
- There should be someone else around so help is nearby if it is needed.
- Use of a baby monitor might make it easier to listen to what is happening in the bathroom while giving some privacy.
- Turning the hot water thermostat down a few degrees will ensure that the water is never too hot.
- Use of temperature-controlled taps means that water runs at a constant temperature.
- Bathroom and toilet doors should open outwards to stop the door being blocked if someone falls behind it

- Use of locks that can be unlocked from outside: this allows privacy but equally means that someone can open the door if need arises.

In the bedroom

Safety pillows

- Safety or 'anti-suffocation' pillows are sometimes used by individuals who have seizures while they are sleeping (nocturnal seizures).
- The safety pillows are ventilated so that if someone is sleeping face down and they have a seizure they should still be able to breathe.

The bed

- If there is a risk of the individual falling out of bed while having a seizure, then low-level beds should be used,
- Futons may help lower the chance of an injury happening.
- Individuals who sleep by themselves may prefer to sleep in the middle of a double bed to reduce falling out of the bed if they have a seizure in their sleep.

In the garden

There are several ways to make the garden a safer place for individual who suffer seizures:

- The type of ground covering should be taken into consideration when laying a lawn which may help reduce the risk of injury if someone falls. Wooden decking instead of stone patio may lower the severity of injury if a person falls.
- Use of a petrol lawn mower instead of electric mower to avoid the risk of a person mowing the cable during a seizure.
- 'Power breaker' plug points are therefore recommended for everyone who uses an electric mower to reduce the risk of electrocution.
- The use of a lawn mower that stops automatically when the handle is released is recommended.

If a garden has a pond

- The pond should be seen from the house or if the pond is being laid it should be visible from the house.
- A fence should be put around the pond to prevent someone from falling into it.
- Cover the pond with a combination of heavy-duty wooden trellis and wire mesh that makes it difficult for someone to fall into it.
- Growing big plants or shrubs around the deeper side of a pond makes it difficult to get close to the edge.
  Fit a safety grid that sits just below the surface of the water which can hold the weight of a person without ruining the look of the pond.

Alarms and monitors

People who live alone and suffer from epilepsy should have alarms and monitors that are triggered when they have a seizure in their sleep (nocturnal seizures).

- Some alarms are triggered when the person is having a seizure.
- Other alarms are triggered by the person when they think they are about to have a seizure.
- The alarms are usually attached to a monitor that prompts instant help.
- The alarms may also be triggered when someone falls down during a seizure.

Outside the home/project

Some people with epilepsy may choose to wear or carry with them something with information that says they have epilepsy.

- National Society of Epilepsy (NSE) produces free identity card which can hold information on:
  - o what type of seizures a person has;
  - o what medication they are taking;
  - o how they can be supported if they are having a seizure.
- Bracelets and necklaces are available which have either a person's medical details or a telephone number where further information can be obtained.
- These can be useful if the person is taken to the hospital as the doctors will quickly be able to obtain information about the epilepsy history and medication they are treated with.
- If the person has communication difficulties and carries with them a communication passport, their medical history on epilepsy should be included.

10.8 Diabetes

10.8.1 What is diabetes?

Diabetes mellitus is a condition in which the amount of glucose (sugar) in the blood is too high because the body cannot use it properly. Glucose comes from the digestion of starchy foods such as:

- bread, rice, potatoes, yams and plantain;
- from sugar;
- other sweet foods;
- from the liver which makes glucose.

Insulin is vital for life. It is a hormone produced by the pancreas that helps the glucose to enter the cells where it is used as fuel by the body.

The main symptoms of untreated diabetes are:

- increased thirst;
- passing urine frequently – especially at night;
- extreme tiredness/fatigue;
- weight loss without trying;
- genital itching;
- regular episodes of thrush;

- blurred vision;
- extreme hunger.

There are two main types of diabetes. These are:

- Type 1 diabetes, also known as insulin dependent diabetes;
- Type 2 diabetes, also known as non insulin dependent diabetes.

10.8.2   Type 1 diabetes

This type develops when the insulin-producing cells in the body have been destroyed and the body is unable to produce any insulin. Insulin is the key that unlocks the door to the body's cells. Once the door is unlocked, glucose can enter the cells where it is used as fuel. In Type 1 diabetes the body is unable to produce any insulin so there is no key to unlock the door and the glucose builds up in the blood.

This type of diabetes usually appears before the age of 40.

Treatment

Type 1 diabetes is treated by insulin.

- All people with Type 1 diabetes will require insulin eventually with diets and regular exercises.
- Insulin cannot be taken in a tablet form, because, being a protein, it would be digested in the stomach before it had any effect.
- Insulin can be given in different ways, via injection, using a syringe, pen device or via an insulin pump.
- The needle is small, as it only needs to be injected under the skin (subcutaneously), either in the stomach, buttocks, thighs or upper arms.
- The insulin is then absorbed into the small blood vessels and arrives in the bloodstream.

Types of insulin

- There are six main types of insulin available in various combinations and they all work in different ways.
- The healthcare team determine the different options available for the service users with diabetes.

10.8.3   Type 2 diabetes

This type of diabetes develops when the body can still make some insulin, but not enough, or when the insulin that is produced does not work properly (known as insulin resistance).

- This type of diabetes usually appears in people over the age of 40, though common in south Asia and African-Caribbean people.
- It often appears after the age of 25.

Type 2 diabetes can be controlled by use of medication – Metformin tablets which can help achieve good blood glucose control.

- Metformin reduces the amount of glucose produced by the liver, making it easier for the muscle cells to accept insulin.
- Because of the way Metformin works, it doesn't lower the blood glucose enough to cause hypoglycemia (a condition where there is too little glucose or sugar in the blood).
- It can help in weight loss with changes to healthy eating.
- Other medication, including insulin injections, may also be required.

Treatment

Type 2 diabetes can be treated by a combination of either:

- diet and exercise;
- diet;
- exercise, tablets (Metformin) and diet;
- exercise and insulin injections.

Aim of treatment

The main aim of treatment for both types of diabetes is to achieve blood glucose and blood pressure levels as near normal as possible. This, together with a healthy lifestyle:

- will help to improve overall well-being;
- will protect against long-term damage to the eyes, kidneys, nerves, heart and major arteries.

10.9   Learning outcomes

Autistic Spectrum Disorder (ASD)

- To provide an understanding of ASD.
- To illustrate a range of theoretical and practical perspectives on this area and the links and contrasts between them.
- To understand the current evidence-based information on ASD and its effects on learning outcomes.
- To understand the importance of consistency in supporting service users with autism.
- To understand information on autism spectrum disorder and its impact on a service user's learning at school/college.
- To develop an understanding of the processes and strategies for effective staff, parents and professionals partnerships.
- To understand specific strategies on how to advocate to support ongoing learning development;

Mental health

- To identify and list common causes and symptoms of de-compensation and relapse as well as appropriate care-giving responses specific to the individual service user.

- To define the terms hallucination and delusion.
- To identify common triggers (including stress) of delusions and hallucinations.
- To identify and demonstrate appropriate intervention strategies with a service user experiencing a delusion or hallucination.
- To accurately document service user behavioural symptoms, interventions, and outcomes.
- To understand how to support recovery of service users at the individual level.

Physical health

Epilepsy

To gain essential understanding regarding:

- what epilepsy is;
- causes of epilepsy;
- types of seizures;
- treatment of epilepsy;
- psychosocial impact of epilepsy;
- what to do when someone has a seizure.

Diabetes

- To demonstrate a basic knowledge of Type 1 and Type 2 diabetes.
- To critically analyse the relationship between risk factors and the complications of diabetes.
- To demonstrate a detailed knowledge and awareness of the physical management and care of a person with diabetes.
- To analyse, apply and interpret evidence from a range of sources to underpin the care and management of diabetes.
- To apply, develop and evaluate care strategies to promote the health and well-being of the person with diabetes.
- To explore and modify care delivery processes in response to the assessment of service users with diabetes.
- To critically analyse the importance of a multi-professional approach to care and reflect systematically on their own role within such a team.

10.10 Framework for reflective practice

- ➤ *Knowledge:*   What have you learnt from reading this chapter?
- ➤ *Skills:*   What do you know, or can do differently now, that you did not/could not do before reading this chapter?
- ➤ *Practices:*   How can you perform a task now better than before?

10.11 References

American Psychiatric Association (1994) *Diagnostic and Statistical Manual of Mental Disorders*. 4th Edition. Washington, DC: American Psychiatric Association

Andresen, R., Oades, L. and Caputi, P. (2003) The experience of recovery from schizophrenia: towards an empirically-validated stage model. *Australian and New Zealand Journal of Psychiatry* **37**: 586–94.

Anthony, W.A. (1993) Recovery from mental illness: the guiding vision of the mental health system in the 1990s. *Psychosocial Rehabilitation Journal* **16**(4), 11–23.

Atkins, R.C., Vernon, M.C. and Eberstein, J.A. (2004) *Atkins Diabetes Revolution: Control Your Carbs to Prevent and Manage Type 2 Diabetes*. New York: HarperCollins US.

Attwood, T. (1998) *Asperger's Syndrome: A Guide for Parents and Professionals.* London: Jessica Kingsley.

Barraclough, N. (2012) *Emergency First Aid Made Easy: A Comprehensive First Aid Manual and Reference Guide.* Qualsafe Ltd.

Bentall, R.P. and Beck, A.T. (2003) *Madness Explained: Psychosis and Human Nature.* Harmondsworth: Penguin

Boutot, E.A. and Tincani, M. (2009) *Autism Encyclopedia: The Complete Guide to Autism Spectrum Disorder*. Woodway, TX: Prufrock Press.

Brooker, C. and Repper, J. (2000) *Serious Mental Health Problems in the Community: Policy, Practice and Research.* Oxford: Bailliere Tindall

Deegan, P. (1988) Recovery: the lived experience of rehabilitation, *Psychosocial Rehabilitation* **11**: 11–19.

Department of Health (1983): Mental Health Act 1983. Code of Practice, chapter 20

Epilepsy Society (2011) Keeping safe inside and outside the home.
http://www.epilepsysociety.org.uk/AboutEpilepsy/Livingwithepilepsy/Epilepsyandsafety

Frith, U. (1989) *Autism and Asperger Syndrome*, Cambridge: Cambridge University Press.

Frith, U. (2008) *Autism: A Very Short Introduction*. Oxford: Oxford University Press.

Gamble, C. and Brennan, G. (2000) *Working with Serious Mental Illness: A Manual for Clinical Practice.* London: Harcourt.

Grandin, T. (2006) *Thinking in Pictures.* London: Bloomsbury.

Hope R. (2004) *The Ten Essential Shared Capabilities – A Framework for the Whole of the Mental Health Workforce.* London: Department of Health

Johnson, J. and Van Rensselaer, A. (2008) *Families of Adults with Autism. Stories and Advice for the Next Generation.* London: Jessica Kingsley.

May, D. (ed.) (2001) *Transition and Change in the Lives of People with Intellectual Disabilities.* London, Jessica Kingsley.

MDF: The Bipolar Organisation. www.mdf.org.uk

Mckernan, T. and Mortlock, J. (2001) *Autism Focus.* St Leonards on Sea: Outset Publishing.

Mencap (2010) *View Point*: Sept/Oct. http://www.mencap.org/gettingitright

Morgan, H. (1996) *Adults with Autism.* Cambridge: Cambridge University Press.

Owen, S. and Saunders, A. (2008) *Bipolar Disorder: The Ultimate Guide.* Oneworld Publication. www.minddisorders.com

Redfield Jamison, K. (1997) *An Unquiet Mind.* New York: Vintage Books. (Kay Redfield Jamison is a psychiatrist who has bipolar disorder.)

Rivera, D.J. (n.d.) Diabetes insipidus: prevention and treatment. ArticleCity.
http://www.articlecity.com/articles/health/article_8531.shtml

Sanofi Aventis (2006) Understanding Type 2 diabetes. Helping make sense of Diabetes. www.sanofi-aventis.co.uk

Scottish Recovery Network (2006) *Journeys of Recovery: Stories of Hope and Recovery from Long Term Mental Health Problems*. Glasgow: Scottish Recovery Network.

Shore S.M. and Rastelli, L.G. (2006) *Understanding Autism for Dummies.* Indianapolis, Indiana: John Wiley & Sons, Inc.

Slade M. (2009a) *100 Ways to Support Recovery: A Guide for Mental Health Professionals*. London: Rethink. www.100_Ways_to_Support_Recovery.pdf

Slade M (2009b) *Personal Recovery and Mental Illness. A Guide for Mental Health Professionals.* Cambridge: Cambridge University Press.

South London and Maudsley NHS Foundation Trust (2007) *Social Inclusion, Rehabilitation and Recovery Strategy 2007–2010*. London: South London and Maudsley NHS Foundation Trust.
Thompson, N. and Thompson, S. (2008) *The Social Work Companion*. London: Palgrave Macmillan.
Williams, D. (1996) *Autism: An Inside Approach*. London: Jessica Kingsley.
Wing, L. (1996) *The Autistic Spectrum: New Updated Edition*. London: Constable & Robinson Ltd.

10.12 Induction workbook

1. What do the terms 'learning disabilities'/'learning difficulties' mean?

   _____
   _____

2. What do you understand by the term 'physical disability'?

   _____
   _____

3.   What does sensory impairment mean? Give examples.

   _____
   _____

4. What do you understand by the term autism?

   _____
   _____

5. Explain the meaning of the term 'mental health' and name the legislation regulating it.

   _____
   _____

6. Why do you think that the service users themselves developed the idea of a social model of disability?

   _____
   _____

7. What do you need to consider about the environment when supporting an individual with ASD?

   _____
   _____

8. List five user-friendly elements of supporting a service user with ASD, taking into consideration communication, organisation and strategy (yourself)

   _____
   _____

9. How will this knowledge help you to support a service user in leading a fulfilling and meaningful life?

    _____

    _____

10. What is the recovery position? Why is it important to put someone who has suffered unconsciousness into the recovery position while they are unconscious?

    _____

    _____

11. What do you understand by the term *Status epilepticus*? What should you do?

    _____

    _____

11   Challenging Behaviour

AIMS

- To create awareness of how challenging behaviours are linked to conditions in learning disabilities especially autistic spectrum disorders

- To understand challenging behaviour as a form of communication

- To provide an overview of how organisations view and manages challenging behaviour

- To understand the role of the multidisciplinary team

11.1   Introduction

There are occasions when service users become angry, frustrated or upset and react in challenging ways, such as showing physical, emotional or verbal aggression.

It is important that you are able to recognise the potential triggers for the individual service user and use developed effective communication skills to prevent challenging situations from arising. It is not always possible to prevent such situations and therefore you need to be equipped with knowledge and skills to address these incidents in the most appropriate way for the service user concerned before they escalate. It is important you understand behaviour that challenges services by asking these questions:

- What is it?
- Why does it happen?
- Who does it challenge?

11.2   Defining challenging behaviour

The term challenging behaviour has been defined as

> culturally abnormal behaviour(s) of such intensity, frequency or duration that the physical safety of the person or others is likely to be placed in serious jeopardy, or behaviour which is likely to seriously limit use of, or result in to a person being denied access to, ordinary community facilities. (Emerson, 1995, pp. 4–5)

To help understand this definition in a layman's language, it will be helpful to break down the main components, which are:

- 'culturally abnormal behaviours' may be defined as behaviours that are disturbing (socially unacceptable), distressing and maladaptive;
- 'safety of self or others being placed in serious jeopardy' – this means people are in danger of being physically hurt and the danger of someone harming themselves or causing emotional distress to self or others;
- 'likely to seriously limit use of, or result in to a person being denied access to, ordinary community facilities'. The behaviour stops the person from being supported to access

activities in the community leading to social exclusion, for example going swimming, lunch out in public restaurants or bowling, thus limiting the person's quality of life.

11.3   Legislation

The policy and accompanying procedures are based on the requirements of the Health and Safety at Work Act 1974, Management of Health and Safety at Work Regulations 1992, the Reporting of Diseases and Dangerous Occurrences Regulations 1995 (RIDDOR 1995) and the Occupiers Liability Act 1957.

It also incorporates the National Minimum Standards from the Care Standards Act 2000, the Domiciliary Care Agencies Regulations 2002.

11.4   Causes of challenging behaviour

11.4.1   Communication factors

Communication difficulties: Being nonverbal, hearing loss, unclear communication, insufficient vocabulary or means of expression, difficulties understanding communication of others and lacking the communication and emotional skills to convey what they need. For people with autism who have no other way to communicate that they are experiencing sensory overload, who are having difficulty with transitions, or who are unable to communicate needs or wants.

11.4.2   Environmental (social and physical) factors

- Environmental factors may contribute to the problem of challenging behaviour where service users may react negatively to noise, heat, and cold or to invasion of their space.
- Some service users, particularly those with autistic spectrum disorders, may be over-sensitive to certain stimuli such as noise, and may therefore react by displaying challenging behaviour.

Other environmental factors include:

- gaining social attention;
- escape or avoidance of demands or social interactions;
- gaining access to preferred activities or objects;
- sensory feedback, e.g. hand flapping, eye poking;
- pursuit of power and control over own life/environment;
- reduction of arousal and anxiety;
- challenging behaviour.

11.4.3   Living and working environment

Important social and physical environmental factors include:

- family background;
- cultural factors or values;
- economic environment;

- school and day-occupation setting;
- type of accommodation;
- rapport with other people in the person's life;
- training and skill of the direct caregivers;
- opportunity for social interactions.

11.4.4 Psychological trauma

- Reaction to abuse
- Bereavement

11.4.5 Medical factors

Medical factors include:

- challenging behaviour may have an underlying medical cause or reason, such as pain or discomfort, illness or sensory difficulties;
- some forms of challenging behaviour are particularly associated with certain conditions and disabilities such as repeated and involuntary body movements (tics) and uncontrollable vocal sounds (Tourette's syndrome) or ritualistic or obsessive behaviour (autistic spectrum disorders);
- substance abuse;
- neuropsychiatric disorders: epilepsy, Tourette's syndrome, attention-deficit hyperactivity disorder (ADHD);
- syndrome-specific conditions and behavioural phenotypes such as Prader-Willi syndrome, Lesch-Nyhan syndrome, Williams syndrome.

11.4.6 Psychiatric factors

Psychiatric factors include:

- depression.
- mood disorders
- schizophrenia

11.5 Warning signs of challenging behaviour

- increased restlessness;
- general body tension;
- irritation;
- withdrawal;
- refusal to communicate/language use (verbalise their thoughts and feelings);
- general over-arousal of body systems (increased breathing and heart rate, muscle twitching etc.);
- pacing;
- increased volume of speech;

- erratic movements;
- thought process unclear;
- poor concentration;
- tense and angry facial expressions.

11.6 Types of challenging behaviour

- physical aggression;
- violent behaviour;
- fire setting;
- inappropriate sexual behaviour;
- self-injurious behaviour (including ingestion or inhalation of foreign bodies);
- withdrawal and isolative behaviour;
- anger;
- self-neglect.

11.7 Functions of challenging behaviour for service users

11.7.1 Attention-seeking behaviour

Attention-seeking behaviour has the purpose of gaining attention from others, either negative or positive. Some service users may be unable to manage a particular task and may be frustrated or bored. However, attention-seeking behaviour can also be a learned behaviour, which has been effective in the past in ensuring that the service users get what they want. Even negative attention can be motivating for some service users, especially if they feel that this is the only attention they can receive.

11.7.2 Other factors

- Gaining/maintaining access to desired item/activity – that is, pursuit of preferred activities without any ability to consider the consequences.
- Escape – escaping/avoiding situations, demands, social interactions.
- Pressure to do tasks that are too difficult or that are disliked or go on for too long.
- Sensory – to provide stimulation.
- Sensory issues – oversensitivity to sensory input/overload from loud sounds, bright lighting, being touched, or too close proximity to other people.
- For some service users smells can be the cause of intense distress and challenging behaviours.

11.8 Triggers of challenging behaviour

- Effecting change in repetitive and ritualistic behaviours, which are important ways of making the world safe to the individual.
- Effecting changes to routines without prior warning.

- Frustration when trying to communicate or not being allowed to speak out or get his/her point across.
- If the service user continues to see challenging behaviour as a means of problem-solving or gaining her/his objective.
- If the service user becomes bored and frustrated.
- If the service user perceives staff are not listening to him/her or not taking his/her unhappiness seriously.
- If the service user becomes angry and resentful towards other service users or staff; this risk is increased if the resentment is about their perception of other people going home for visits, having boyfriends or their sisters having children and starting a family.
- Strong expectations being placed upon a service user and lack of recognition at how well they are doing.

11.9 Guidelines for working with people with challenging behaviour

Social care workers should at all times understand they have a legal duty to their safety first, their colleagues, people they support and visitors from their actions or omissions. Therefore, it is essential that all staff supporting someone with challenging behaviour should know:

- how to work safely and properly with the person taking into account:

  o the person's communication potential/style;
  o the person's patterns of communication – verbal, written, sign, symbols or objects; are you (staff) able to understand them?
  o are the resources needed to achieve their understanding available? (training, risk assessment, guidelines, etc.)
  o is the person allowed to make informed choices?
  o does the person have access to support and does he/she feel supported?

- the reporting procedures – recording information – how? by ticking charts, recording sheets and Antecedent – Behaviour – Consequences (ABC) charts, which helps:

  o to look for patterns in behaviour;
  o understand when it is happening;
  o why the individual engages in problem behaviour.

Once the function or purpose of a pattern of behaviour is identified, it is then possible to design interventions directly targeting the underlying reason for why it occurs.

11.9.1 Incident forms

Where a problem arises related to aggression and violence in the work situation, staff must fill in an incident/accident form detailing the circumstances of any incident of challenging behaviour or aggression which has taken place. Documentation will help all parties when evaluating re-occurring incidents.

Incident records are descriptions of specific events, such as when a person engages in an incident of challenging behaviour e.g., kicking another service user, punching staff, absconding. While incident records describe the challenging behaviour, e.g., when it occurred, how intense it was, and what happened as a result, they do not describe anything other than the specific event). It is therefore, important to fill out an A-B-C chart.

11.9.2   A–B-C chart (antecedent–behaviour–consequences form)

- Antecedents – descriptions of events/situation in details prior to the incident including location of other service users and staff if relevant.
- Behaviours – descriptions of behaviours exhibited
- Consequences and response to behaviour – description in details of action and words of staff and of physical (i.e. deflection, breakaway, and escort with reference to physical intervention policy if applicable) and/ or non-physical intervention techniques used (i.e. active listening, empathy, negotiation, distraction)

11.9.3   Other steps to take following an incident/accident

- Inform the home/project/residential manager at the earliest stage.
- All staff must adhere to any advice, procedures or systems introduced in order to reduce or eliminate risk identified in the risk assessment.
- Ensure that staff are supported, e.g. debriefing and counselling for post-traumatic stress and fear resulting from an incident of challenging behaviour.

11.9.4   The role of the service manager

The service managers with the assistance from staff should:

- carry out a risk assessment of each work situation, taking into account the individual being supported, the environment where the support is provided and furnishing that have the potential to be used as weapons on the staff;
- take all necessary measures to eliminate risks found and where this is not achievable to reduce the risks to the lowest level practical as stipulated in the Health and Safety at Work Act 1974;
- ensure that all staff who would be working with the individual have received appropriate training and are up to date with conflict management and physical intervention techniques;
- advise all employees of the risks to health and how these are to be avoided;
- in the circumstances where staff raise a matter related to aggression and violence, steps should be taken to investigate the situation and take corrective measures where appropriate; this may mean revising the risk assessments and procedures;
- advise staff of actions taken and records kept in regards to:

  o   the risk assessments;
  o   action taken as a result of the risk assessments;
  o   information shared with staff;

 o action taken in respect to incidents;
 o training – who has been trained and in what;

- have the behaviour support plan in place for all staff working with service users with challenging behaviour which:

 o staff will follow to provide individual support strategies aimed at reducing the incidence of challenging behaviour;
 o specifies the graded response needed to safeguard service users who challenge services through their behaviour;
 o describes individual primary and secondary prevention strategies and the safe and effective use of restrictive physical interventions;
 o describes the primary prevention strategies necessary to meet the complex support needs of service users with learning disabilities and autism that will prevent challenging behaviour;
 o describes the secondary preventions strategies that will distract or de-escalate a situation at an early stage that has the potential to escalate into an episode of challenging behaviour.

11.10 Person-centred guidelines to prevent challenging behaviour

Challenging behaviour should never be considered to be mere attention-seeking, as there are always reasons for it. Every behaviour serves a purpose, especially for children/adults with ASD, either to communicate, to relieve anxiety, to self-stimulate, to exert control over his/her environment, to escape or to avoid, among other things.

The first priority for staff is to prevent a challenging situation from either occurring or worsening. Here are ways to help prevent incidents of challenging behaviour.

- Acting to diffuse a challenging situation at its earliest stage.
- Reviewing the lifestyle, health and environment of the person being supported.
- Monitoring and revising a reasonably coherent plan for providing support to service users which takes into account:

 o the triggers;
 o altering the antecedents of the behaviour, e.g. filling the individual's time more meaningfully;
 o specific procedures for reducing challenging behaviour such as de-escalation.

- Managing one's own behaviour appropriately, including the team working in a consistent approach.

Support staff should consider how best to provide the most effective possible opportunities for an individual to communicate their feelings in all aspect of their lives.

According to Emerson (1995), 'Challenging behaviour is often an individual's communication about dissatisfaction with their physical or social environment or the nature of the support being provided.'

11.11 What staff should do when challenging behaviour happens

11.11.1 Responding to behaviour

How to make decision

- The strategy used to managing an incident so that the likelihood of a safe outcome is achieved should be individualised.
- The first step should be to identify what is already known about the specific support that helps to keep the individual and others safe.
- The techniques that diffuse escalation and things that help when the individual is at the verge of losing control or has lost control.

Once an incident is under way there are a number of possible ways to deal with it. The techniques listed below are not separate from each other and are often used in combination, according to situation and the behaviour support plan of the service user.

- Planned ignoring – there are times when non-action has a limiting effect on behaviour. One option of dealing with an incident is to do absolutely nothing and allow events to run their course without any active intervention. The skill is in knowing when to intervene and when not to.
- Clear the area – move away from the person, and remove others (audience) and let the individual calm down in their own time.
- Call for physical support – if there is access to other staff at the home or project or specialist crisis support team that can be called out to help. (In most medium/high secure/ treatment units or hospitals, there are usually response teams that respond to calls for physical support.) Alternatively staff should call the police for assistance, especially if lone working.
- Move the person – physically move the person to a safe area and let them calm down at their own time. This is for extreme situations where violence is used or threatened and removal is the safest solution, by two trained members of staff or calling in the police.
- Stay with the person – this involves remaining present and using breakaway techniques to maintain safety; for example, breaking away from bites, grabs to the body or clothes.
- Restraining the person – this would involve either holding specific limbs, e.g. their hands in front of them or more generally restraining the individual's body until they have calmed down, and is usually performed by two trained staff.
- Call for advisory support – there should be access to an on-call support service that should work with staff in terms of providing emotional support and guidance on the management of the incident in progress.

Caution: Under no circumstances should staff intervene if an individual has a weapon. '*A weapon can be any object with an applied threat to use offensively.*' Staff should make the area safe, withdraw and call the police for assistance.

When faced with a challenging situation staff should:

- appear calm and confident;

- be aware of a safe exit;
- speak clearly and calmly with a firm tone of voice;
- clearly state what is required;
- focus on behaviour, not the person;
- don't be challenging or aggressive;
- have confidence in your behaviour management skills;
- consider previous episodes of challenging behaviour;
- recognise positive behaviour and praise it;
- remain relaxed and breath normally;
- maintain comfortable eye contact but do not stare;
- keep movements slow and composed – quick actions may surprise and scare the other person.

11.11.2 Effective ways of dealing with challenging and inappropriate behaviour

Service users may not understand that it is their behaviour that triggers the system of consequences and that it should be brought to their attention. Staff should aid appropriate behaviour by:

- maintaining a clear, consistent and reasonable approach from all staff; it is essential in order to be successful and non-damaging to the therapeutic relationship with the service user;
- recognising and acting on the need for accurate observation and assessment of behaviour before change can occur;
- recognising and acting on the need for a flexible and individual approach to each service user and behaviour;
- when attempting to change behaviour/routine, it is important that collaborative assessment is conducted; this will help to avoid the service user's existing behaviour being replaced by more challenging behaviour;
- nurturing a positive view of the self, by demonstrating compassion in their response to a service user who reports setbacks, for example in self-harming;
- accentuating positive behaviour in a service user because:

  o it focuses on a service user's positive behaviour rather than their challenging behaviour;
  o it minimises the response to challenging behaviour and highlights the response to positive behaviour; however, it is important not to ignore challenging behaviour especially when people's safety could be at risk;
  o it encourages positive behaviour to be repeated and strengthens the relationship between the carer and the service user;
  o it enables staff to model appropriate behaviour;
  o it promotes a more rewarding and motivating environment for both staff and service users;
  o it provides the service users with clear information about what is acceptable and appropriate.

11.12 Management and strategies of challenging behaviour

11.12.1 Multidisciplinary team (MDT)

The multidisciplinary team (MDT) is a group of professionals who work side-by-side to provide a holistic approach, ensuring individuals are provided with a coordinated service. Assessment and treatment approaches are tailored to meet the needs of each individual and support successful outcomes.

The MDT may include any two of the following: psychologists, speech and language therapist (SALT), psychiatrics and other health professionals in collaboration with the staff, to provide clear and accurate information regarding the management of the service user.

Multidisciplinary teams, in collaboration with the care teams, develop behaviour support plans to provide caregivers and staff with a comprehensive set of strategies aimed at both reducing and managing occurrences of challenging behaviour and promoting growth and skills development (e.g. communication, or social skills etc.), for service users with challenging behaviours.

Behaviour support plans are developed by analysing the service user's challenging behaviour in routines, activities, and/or interactions with others, in relation to internal factors (including learning disabilities and effect like autistic spectrum disorders) and external factors (i.e. environmental, communication etc.)

11.12.2 The elements of a user friendly support plan

- A support plan is the document that staff will follow to provide individual support strategies aimed at reducing the incidence of challenging behaviour.
- A support plan is a care plan that specifies the graded response needed to safeguard service users who challenge services through their behaviour.
- A support plan describes individual primary and secondary prevention strategies and the safe and effective use of restrictive physical interventions.
- A support plan describes the primary prevention strategies necessary to meet the complex support needs of service users with learning disabilities and autism that will prevent challenging behaviour.
- A support plan describes the secondary preventions strategies that will distract or de-escalate a situation at an early stage that has the potential to escalate into an episode of challenging behaviour.

11.13 Strategies of intervention to help manage challenging behaviour

11.13.1 Structure

The structure of interventions simply identifies what staff plans to do.

- It is a summary of the team's decision on which strategy will be done. Where appropriate, it should also identify who is going to implement the strategy, and where and when it will be done.

- The focus is on what team members will do rather than on what the service user will do. Exceptions to this occur when the service user is part of the planning process. However, one should not confuse a contract with a Behaviour Intervention Plan.

11.13.2 Process

The process describes how something is done. When working with service users who have emotional/behavioural disorders, the success or failure of an intervention strategy can depend as much on how something is done as what is done. Once a team member realises that an intervention must be done in a certain way to be successful, it is important to share this with the team. This will help other caregivers implement the intervention more effectively.

11.14 Prevention strategies

Prevention strategies include the responses that caregivers and professionals provide or the alterations that may be made to an environment that make challenging behaviour irrelevant (Hieneman *et al.*, 1999).

11.14.1 Diffusing

In a care setting, should a challenging situation occur, there are a number of techniques and approaches that can be used to diffuse the situation as outlined in the behaviour support plan. However, it is essential that an approach is not used without having it agreed as part of an individual support plan by the multidisciplinary care team.

The following are some techniques that can be used to diffuse a situation.

1. *Deflecting*

Staff can deflect the situation by encouraging the concerned service user to focus on a different task or situation. Doing something different changes the focus of a person's attention and prevents the situation from escalating.

2. *Comforting*

Staff may seek to comfort the person verbally and if appropriate, by gentle physical contact. It is important that touching is appropriate and that professional boundaries should be considered. Some people with ASD do not like to be touched and may react adversely

3. *Reinforcing positive behaviour*

- Reinforcing positive behaviour is part of the Behaviour Support Plan approach, which seeks to understand the function of a service user's challenging behaviour and then works with them to reduce or remove the need for that behaviour to occur.
- Staff should try to empower the service user in finding alternative coping strategies they may find helpful and focus on positive aspects that may help to build their self-esteem.
- Staff should let the service users know they have choices.
- Use reward approach appropriately, with praise or attention for any positive behaviour the person may be showing, there is need to identify the reinforcers that are meaningful to the

person. For instance when coping with unstructured times and waiting at the GPs surgery, staff should communicate to the individual how well they have done and 'treat' them on the way back home as a reward.

4. *Personal space*

Staff should offer the person some lone time, suggesting going to a quiet place away from the existing environment, for example to their bedroom or flat to listen to music. Or sensory room where there are recreational facilities.

5. *Silence*

Silence is one of the most effective verbal intervention techniques. Silence on the part of staff allows the individual to clarify and restate the problem. This often leads to clear understanding of the true source of the individual's conflict.

11.14.2 Self-management

When people come to work, sometimes they bring their emotional baggage and moods with them and the impact of this should never be understated. It is important, therefore, that:

- every member of staff should have a positive approach when at work;
- staff work as a team to provide a consistent approach; all staff should be clear and keep giving the same message;
- staff should have time to reflect on their own feelings, as working with service users with challenging behaviour can evoke strong emotions.

11.14.3 Verbal de-escalation technique

- Verbal de-escalation techniques are part of secondary prevention strategy which is nonphysical skills combined with effective communication used to prevent a potentially dangerous situation from escalating into a physical confrontation.
- There are three clear phases in the management of challenging behaviour. These are: the calming phase, when a decision has been made to respond or intervene in an incident of challenging behaviour, the staff member dealing with the incident must try to instil some calm into the proceedings by demonstrating their own ability to stay calm, which will calm the individual and hopefully lead to a building of some rapport and allow them (staff) to find a satisfactory solution to the source of the problem.

1. *The calming phase*

- In order to begin to de-escalate a difficult situation, staff have to first instil an element of calm by allowing the service user some space and moving back or changing position. When someone is agitated or stressed it may be necessary to give them more space than normal to reassure them that staff (you) are not invading their personal space.
- When the service user steps forward and invades the personal space of a staff member, getting uncomfortably close, it may be advisable to step back and re-establish their

personal space. Staff should open their posture and adopt a non-threatening and non-defensive posture, by standing slightly to the side and keeping their hands open with space between them and the service user. Staff should be assertive in their communication by controlling their voice, maintaining an even tone and pitch and speaking slowly and clearly.

2. *Building rapport*

- Staff builds rapport when they listen to what the service user is saying, and showing that they are listening by reflecting back the important parts of what has been said, asking open-ended questions that do not require a simple yes/no answer. Open-ended questions ask the person to think and reflect, give opinions and express their feelings. This will engage them in a constructive conversation (see Chapter 2, Section 2.14, Verbal skills to overcome communication barriers, p. 59).
- Explaining things clearly and giving reasons where appropriate and always ensuring ample time and opportunity are given to the service user to answer. Staff should always seek a common ground before moving on to more contentious issues, and where appropriate offer an apology, and invite the service user to offer suggestions as to how to resolve any disagreement. It is important that staff empathise and show understanding, trying to see things from their (service user's) point of view.
- Establish the cause: There may have been a genuine reason for being angry and sometimes all is needed is an acknowledgement of this. In case there is any deadlock, staff may consider making a concession, some form of token gesture that shows that they are willing to yield first. However, staff should always avoid giving ultimatums or threats instead offer choices. People like to feel in control.

3. *Reaching a positive solution*

Once staff (where the situation is being dealt with on a one-to-one basis) have engaged the service user in constructive dialogue, where appropriate, begin to work with them (service user) towards an appropriate conclusion in order to bring about a sense of closure to an incident by summarising what has happened including an outline of any agreed plan of action and timeframes. It is important that this is communicated to the team members.

- If despite your best efforts the service user is not calming down – or even may be escalating the situation with you – it might be worthwhile to consider asking if it would be better to get another staff member to deal with the situation, especially if you are perceived by the service user as part of the problem, in which case your continuing presence may not be helping.
- Whenever there is a positive outcome, always thank the service user for their co-operation, even if you don't get back a civil response from them.

4. *Proactive strategies*

Proactive strategies aim to reduce the occurrence of risk/challenging behaviours or prevent them from occurring in the first place. They might include:

- increasing social activities identified as relevant to the person to reduce boredom and therefore reduce the risks of self injury/aggression towards staff;
- providing someone with psychological therapy to help them understand why they are angry and upset after, for example, a failed home visit due to unforeseen circumstances with the parents/guardians.

Proactive strategy is therefore, the first step towards a positive interaction that could build trust. The purpose of proactive strategies is to identify and design interventions based on our understanding of the service user, his/her personal/emotional programming needs, so the service user does not have to use his/her survival strategies to cope with everyday situations.

There are several proactive strategies designed to help manage challenging behaviour. These are management guidelines set out in conjunction with the multidisciplinary team.

- collaborative problem solving and risk assessment;
- daily behaviour rating scales;
- social stories;
- behaviour contracts;
- traffic lights system;
- reward charts;
- verbal de-escalation.

11.14.4 Collaborative problem-solving

Collaborative problem solving, devised by Drs Ross Greene and Stuart Albon, is defined as :

> A process by which adults and kids resolve problems together when they approach problems collaboratively and work toward solutions that are mutually satisfactory, things head in a positive direction. It's very hard work, but it's a lot better than the alternative. This can be achieved through negotiations. (Greene, 2005)

The main purposes of collaborative problem solving are:

- recognising that the service user's behaviour is a result of their own difficulties;
- it discourages clients from being seen as a 'manipulative', 'attention-seeking', 'bad' or 'playing up';
- it focuses upon teaching the individual the skills they lack, e.g. communication through sign language, symbols or objects of reference/picture, gesture, body language and facial expressions.

11.14.5 Collaborative risk assessments

These are risk assessment completed collaboratively with the service user, the psychologist, staff and information from previous notes. They play an important role in that:

- it allows staff to be aware of the potential triggers that may lead to incidents of self-injurious behaviour, suicide, and physical aggression;

- it identifies factors that decrease the risk of these behaviours being demonstrated;
- involving more staff in drawing the risk assessment gives a better coverage for spotting risks from a wide range of sources;
- it creates a greater risk-awareness culture throughout the care environment;
- the more people involved in collaborative risk assessment the better since they can see the potential problems and triggers and have ideas about potential solutions;
- giving staff the opportunity to propose solutions, carry them out and see the benefits, is a good motivator which boosts morale beyond risk management activities;
- collaborative risk assessment allows the line manager to manage the process, check progress and changes, support proactive solutions and ensure that they are implemented, rather than being swamped or even ignored.

11.14.6 Daily Behaviour Rating Scale

The Daily Behaviour Rating Scale (DBRS) is a tool that can be used to monitor a service user's behaviour. The DBRS can be structured and tailored to meet the assessment needs of any individual, and may be implemented for a short- or long-term period.

How the Daily Behaviour Rating Scale works

- A definition of the behaviour to be monitored (for example, physical aggression or self-injurious behaviour) must be agreed before staff begin rating the behaviour.
- It is staff's responsibility to record when there are indicators of the behaviour to be rated (this is rated as 'a definite indication', 'some indication', and 'no indication').

For instance, if staff were monitoring a service user's aggressive behaviour, they would first agree a definition of the behaviour to be monitored (e.g. physical violence towards another service user or object). 'A definite indication' might be punching another person, and 'no indication' would be when the service user did not demonstrate any indicators at all of the behaviour being monitored.

The Daily Behaviour Rating Scale must be reviewed regularly to ensure:

- it is being completed accurately;
- it is effectively achieving its assessment aims;
- and that action may be taken as necessary in response to the service user's behaviour.

11.14.7 Social stories

Carol Gray defines social stories as vignettes of social etiquette 'designed to explain how social interactions work, with the basis of reinforcing appropriate behaviour' (Gray and McAndrew, 2001). They are short written stories to help the service user understand a small part of their social world and behave appropriately within it.

Social stories contain directives, descriptive, affirmative and perspective sentences.

- Directive sentences are used to suggest appropriate actions and instruct how to decode recognition. An example of a directive sentence: 'I will get on my pyjamas at 9.00 pm, so that I will be ready for bed at 10 pm.' The expected behaviour is to be in bed at 10 pm. The behaviour that will lead to the expected end is to have pyjamas on at 9.00 pm.

- Affirmative sentences are used to express commonly shared values or opinions of people in a given situation. An example of an affirmative sentence: 'It is good to listen to your key worker.'
- Descriptive sentences aid understanding about: Who? What? When? Where? Why? How? These are the indisputable facts about a situation or setting or people. They are logical and accurate, factual statements summarising the situation. An example of a descriptive sentence: 'We go for a gardening session every Thursday at 11.00 am.'
- Perspective sentences are used to describe the thoughts and feelings of other people. Occasionally perspective sentences may be used to describe or refer to the internal state of a person with an autistic spectrum disorder, e.g. 'The team leader is happy when I attend all my day's activities.'

Importance of social stories as a communication tool

- Each social story provides clear, concise and accurate information about what is happening in a specific social situation, outlining why it is happening and what a typical response might be in that social situation.
- Each social story aims to provide answers to key questions about a social situation that is problematic to the service user.
- An effective social story can enable a person to revisit the same social situation regularly, and remind them of their personal role in that social situation.
- Social stories are equally beneficial to staff because they learn to deal with and alter the way they deal with difficult social situations.
- They help staff develop more awareness that they are often a part of the problem, not just the answer.

The process of developing the story increases social understanding for both the person with ASD and the person supporting those with Autistic Spectrum Disorders.

11.14.8 Behaviour contract

Behaviour contracts are written to help service users feel secure and supported in their attempts to change their behaviour and improve their quality of interaction.

Importance of behaviour contracts

- They can serve to alleviate anxiety by offering a clear and consistent approach to an ongoing problem.
- They are written to benefit the service user above anyone else and so the service user must be involved in the writing of the entire contract.
- For the contracts to be effective, they are not to be done *for* the service users, they are to be done *with* them.

Outline the reason for the contract

- This part should give a brief explanation as to the current behaviour/situation.
- It should explain why the behaviour/situation occurs, why it needs to change and what the benefit of the change will be.
- It should be written purely to clarify the situation and should not have any negative language. No blame should be attributed.
- Explanations must be clear and written in a language a service user can understand.

Wording of the contract

The Service user agrees that:

- List the behaviour the service user will try to do.
- This must be realistic and reflect the service user's abilities.
- Setting a service user up to fail by imposing too strict or unachievable guidelines will only distress the service user and have negative consequences for the therapeutic relationship.
- The contract should reflect the environment they are in as well as what would happen if they were living independently in the community.
- Should the service user fail to stick to the contract the consequences should be realistic and never negative.

Signed_____ Dated_____

Staff agrees that:

- List here the things that *all* staff are going to do to support the service user in keeping to their contract.
- This may mean changing current practices if it is having a detrimental effect on the service user.
- It should not include promises which cannot be kept, i.e. It will never be noisy on the project/ward/house ever again. If staff cannot keep to their side of the contract why should the service user?
- It should not give the impression that one service user's needs will be placed over another's and should remain balanced.

Signed on behalf of all staff_____
Job Title_____ Dated_____

11.14.9 Traffic lights system: red, orange and green

The traffic lights system is a way to monitor negative behaviour, while providing a visual reminder of the immediate goal.

What service user means when they say they are on RED

- Service user identifies RED as meaning they feel aggressive or anxious for the following reasons:
  o feeling depressed
  o feeling highly anxious about their situation
  o experiencing low self-esteem
  o doubting their own ability to make things better for themselves.

What are the triggers of RED *to a service user?*

1. staff accusing a service user of attention seeking;
2. feeling under-supported by staff;
3. feeling guilty about an earlier incident, e.g. slamming doors, attacking staff etc.;
4. noisy residential settings;
5. other service users behaviour, i.e. being aggressive or violent;
6. strong expectations being placed on them.

How staff can support a service user in RED

It has been found that where staff are less blaming towards residents, they are more likely to offer more effective support (Dilworth, 2000)

Staff are to treat the service user in the same manner as when on green but with the addition of the following increased support:

- Staff to support the service user through gentle motivation to complete simple, achievable tasks such as making the bed, tidying the flat after breakfast, going for a short walk in the garden.
- The staff should work collaboratively with the service user to help identify possible self-injurious tools. Service users work very well at identifying these and handing them over to staff, if reassured that they will only be kept until they are feeling better.
- Staff should offer one-to-one time to discuss any concerns or issues. It is important that a service user feels they are being listened to and supported.
- Psychologist to engage with the service user to develop self-soothe techniques. Staff will then be informed of the techniques and need to give gentle encouragement to complete them.
- Staff to nurture a positive view of the self, by demonstrating compassion in their response to a service user who reports setbacks

What service user means when they are on GREEN

Service users identify **GREEN** as meaning that s/he is not having active thoughts of aggressiveness. This does not mean a service user is not having difficulties but rather that s/he is currently able to cope effectively, with continual staff support.

What the service user will try to do

- S/he will try to talk to staff about how s/he is feeling before the mood escalates.

- S/he will try to stick to their contract.
- S/he will try and treat others on the project in the same way they would like to be treated themselves.
- Service user will try and be supported to stick to their care plan.

What staff will do to support

- Staff should speak to the service user with empathy and respect.
- Staff to abide by all the service user's care plans, contracts and guidelines in place to maintain consistence.
- Service users often feel frustrated when trying to communicate their point of view. Staff can assist by giving them plenty of time to talk and not interrupt when speaking.
- Service users like to be spoken to clearly and politely. They have difficulty processing lots of information and adapting to new ideas if they are different to how they were expecting them to be. Staff can use visual aids for better clarification of information

It is important for staff to remember that a diagnosis may mean that the service users will need continual support in all areas of their care. It can also mean that the service users' moods may change rapidly and so will require close observation at all times.

11.14.10 Rewarding positive behaviour

- Acknowledge and praise the service user's positive behaviour, for example waiting at the GP's surgery with unstructured times.
- Engage with the service user when they are behaving appropriately.
- Ask questions (e.g. how did you manage to stay calm?) to acknowledge the service user's positive behaviour and encourage them to reflect on successful strategies.
- Talk positively to the service user rather than negatively. Rather than emphasising what they are doing incorrectly, highlight how they can modify their behaviour to make it acceptable.
- Use reward charts: every good behaviour and task achieved earns the service user a 'star'/sticker that represents a reward.

11.14.11 Training: proactive intervention techniques

Skill are required to handle behaviours that are out of control, which will help keep staff safe, help keep the service user safe, and de-escalate the situation.

Some examples of training organisations:

Non Abusive Psychological and Physical Intervention (NAPPI) Website: www.nappiuk.com

Sample: Individual physical intervention policy for John:

    Name: John

    Staffing level **2:1** in doors **3:1** in the Community

    General description and nature of challenging behaviour

- Hitting and kicking fellow service users without warning or sign of agitation
- Damaging property, e.g. kicking stationery vehicles
- Being aggressive towards babies and children especially when they cry

Methods that should be used to de-escalate situations before a physical intervention is needed for John:

- All the staff working with John should read and sign all support guidelines and risk assessments. By signing, the staff agree that they have read and understood them.
- When John shows sign of agitation or becomes verbally aggressive, staff should position themselves between him and an exit so that they are not blocked in a room, making themselves more vulnerable to physical attack.
- Staff should ask other people to move away if possible. Remove the source of John's anxiety if possible.
- Staff should address John by name, communicate effectively with him using his style of communication (verbal), informing him what is required or attempt to redirect him or resolve that issue that has upset him.
- Where necessary or appropriate, staff should withdraw to another part of the house or room that has more than one exit, this is to keep themselves safe to allow John time on his own to calm down.
- Depending on the history of the incident and the risk assessment, PRN medication should be administered as per directions, staff should not leave 'things' until it's too late.
- If John is out in the community, staff should support him to return home as soon as is possible or where the behaviour is a threat to the members of the public, staff should sought police assistance in returning him back home. Staff should not wait until an incident has happened.

Elements of user friendly de-escalation techniques

Staff should be able to identify and understand behaviour and respond appropriately. Behaviour is both purposeful and learned. All behaviour has meaning. First establish the state the person is in. Consider:

1. Is the individual hungry?
2. Is he/she thirsty?
3. Is he/she tired?
4. Is he/she in pain?
5. Is he/she bored or lonely?
6. Does he/she feel supported?

A person does something in order to meet a need or desire. If that need or desire is met, the person is more likely to repeat the behaviour the next time the situation arises.

'Do's and 'don'ts of intervention

Do's

✓ Recognise the triggers and the early warning signs; note the particular circumstances that were occurring at the time. Observe the environment, what was happening, what was being said, noise levels, distractions, or anything else that may have been happening and may have provoked the reaction in the individual.

✓ Know how best to work with potentially difficult, aggressive individuals, what works to keep them safe. Be alert to multiple sources of danger and your exit (risk assessments, care plans and behaviour support plans).

✓ Try and establish a rapport and focus on the working relationship you are trying to create. Focus on the behaviour not the individual.

✓ Attitude: How you behave will have a direct, and often profound, influence on how things turn out. Being calm will instil calmness and help the person to be calm. Reduce stimuli by removing audience or source of anxiety where possible.

✓ Manage and influence the situation; don't attempt to control the person. The person is attempting to be in control. Redirect and negotiate. Communicate understanding and be supportive.

Don'ts

Don't blame, criticise or yell at the individual or move too quickly or with force, or engage in any inappropriate interventions. The person might expect to be criticised or blamed for their behaviour, whatever, their expectations you should affirm their courage by saying something like 'I'm impressed you calmed yourself quickly. Praising the person's demonstration of responsibility increases their confidence.'

Don't assume you know what the person is feeling and what motivates them. You may, and again, you may not. Mistaken assumptions can hurt you, others or the individual.

11.15 Reactive strategies

Reactive strategies are an immediate or emergency response to the risk/challenging behaviour which aims to minimise its intensity. Even with careful planning and effective proactive interventions, service users with severe emotional/behavioural difficulties will get into difficulty. Their problem behaviours are driven by survival or organic issues and, at some point, these will be triggered.

The purposes of reactive strategies are:

- to assist the service user to move out of destructive psychological states where survival strategies can be easily triggered;
- to help the service user return to a more competent psychological state where s/he can gain rational control over emotions and behavioural responses;
- to minimize the disruption to and distressing of others;
- to assist others in feeling safe.

In addition, we may want to take some actions that allow the service user to learn from the incident and assist them in making better choices next time. In some cases where the service user's behaviours place others in danger and when their psychological state makes it difficult for them to respond to reasonable direction or staff control, it may be necessary to develop a safety plan.

11.15.1 Types of reactive strategies

- physical intervention/restraint;
- mechanical restraint;
- administration of Pro Ra Nate (PRN) medication .

11.15.2 Physical intervention/restraint

Physical intervention is a reactive strategy used in management of challenging behaviour; it is a set of nationally recognised restraint techniques for safely managing physical aggression when all attempts at diffusion (proactive) or prevention have failed.

All physical interventions should adhere to local policy, national guidelines and law (DoH, 2002) and be agreed in consultation with the multidisciplinary team, the service user and the supporting staff.

The British Institute for Learning Disabilities describes physical intervention in relation to challenging behaviour as:

> A method of responding to the challenging behaviour of people with learning disability and/or autism which involves some degree of direct physical force which limits or restricts the movement or mobility of the person concerned. (Harris *et al.*, 1996)

11.15.3 Three types of physical intervention

- Direct physical contact between a member of staff and a service user. For example, holding a person's arms and legs to stop them attacking someone (hitting and kicking).
- The use of barriers such as locked doors to limit freedom of movement. For example, placing door catches or bolts beyond the reach of service users.
- Materials or equipment that restricts or prevents movement. For example, placing splints on a person's arms to restrict movement.

Physical intervention should be seen as an absolute last resort and should only be employed by two trained members of staff during emergency situations, for the shortest possible time and should involve reasonable application of minimum force.

11.15.4 Circumstances for using physical intervention

Physical intervention techniques are only for the use by trained staff when there is:
- significant risk of physical assault;
- a serious degree of urgency and danger;
- significant threats or attempts at self-injury;
- risk of serious accidents to self or others.

There are likely to be four main reasons for the use of physical intervention procedures:

(a) The person is actually causing injury to him or herself, which if not stopped, will seriously damage his or her health.
(b) The person is significantly assaulting, or attempting to assault others, to such intensity that injuries will be incurred unless stopped immediately.
(c) The person is causing severe disruption, which, if not intercepted, may lead to a more serious incident occurring.
(d) The person is causing serious environmental damage to objects or property in an environment not specifically designated as their own, which, if not responded to, may result in injury or conflict with another person, a member of the public or harm to themselves or others.

Physical intervention, however, *must never* be used as a form of punishment.

11.15.5 Decision to use physical intervention

- In any situation the decision to intervene will require staff to exercise judgement and discretion about the level of risk. This decision will often need to be taken quickly, based on the likely outcome of not intervening.
- Staff deciding to intervene are expected to take decision with colleagues, taking into account of all the circumstances, including any known history of other events involving the individual to be restrained and to remain respectful of the person and other service user throughout.
- In making the decision to intervene individual guidelines agreed in advanced by a multidisciplinary team, should be followed unless no individual policy exist or the behaviour and the risk had not previously presented itself.
- The scale and nature of any physical intervention must be proportionate to both the behaviour of the individual to be restrained, and the nature of the harm they might cause either to themselves or to others.
- The minimum necessary force should be used, and the techniques deployed should be those with which the staff involved are familiar with (trained) and able to use safely and are described in the service user's support plan

11.15.6 Physical intervention – risk assessment

When the use of a restrictive physical intervention is sanctioned, it is important that the appropriate steps are taken to minimise the risk to both the staff and service users. Particularly when supporting the service user to the floor and using holding techniques to contain them there.

The main risk to the service user is that physical intervention may:
- cause injury;
- be used unnecessarily, that is when other less intrusive methods could achieve the desired outcome;
- cause pain, distress or psychological trauma;
- become routine rather than exceptional methods of management;
- increase the risk of abuse;

- create distrust and undermine personal relationship;
- undermine the dignity of the staff or service users or otherwise humiliate or degrade those involved.

The main risks to staff include the following:
- as a result of applying physical intervention they may suffer injury;
- they may experience distress or psychological trauma;
- they may face legal action for the use of physical intervention if challenged in a court of law in case of death/injuries sustained by the service user;
- disciplinary action is taken for inappropriate or unjustified use of physical interventions when other less intrusive methods could have achieved the desired outcome.

The main risk of not intervening:
- service users, staff or other people could be injured or abused;
- staff may be in breach of the duty of care, i.e. reasonable measures have not been taken to prevent harm;
- serious damage to property could occur;
- the possibility of litigation in respect to these matters.

11.15.7 Mechanical restraint

Mechanical restraint is a device used on a person to restrict free movement. The purpose of a mechanical restraint is to prevent a person from inflicting serious self-injuries, for example wearing splints to prevent bites on the arms or poking their eyes or pulling their hair out.

11.15.8 Administering Pro Ra Nate (PRN) medication

Medication administered to help a person calm down when they are angry. This is given as a last result when all attempts at diffusion (proactive) or prevention have failed.

11.15.9 Cautions regarding reactive strategies

Reactive strategies should always:

- be reviewed at regular specified intervals or whenever necessary;
- be the least restrictive possible intervention;
- use approved and accredited techniques;
- follow best practice and professional guidelines;
- be explained to the person in an accessible format where possible, i.e. subject to their legal capacity, age and understanding.

11.15.10   Types of physical intervention techniques

1. *Breakaway techniques*

Breakaway techniques are exactly what they say, that is breaking/moving away from a situation whereby someone is being verbally and or physically aggressive.

- Techniques range from stepping away from the person being aggressive, to releasing yourself from being held by them and putting distance/space between you.
- On several occasions physical intervention can be avoided by staff using recognised breakaway techniques. For example, there may be times when a staff member is being verbally/physically assaulted but feels that using physical intervention may be too extreme or they are lone working, in supported living services. On these occasions and/or in preparation to using physical intervention, it may be appropriate to use breakaway techniques

2. *Personal space*

In order to support an individual to become calm themselves or to lessen the length of time that physical intervention is used on them, the individual may be encouraged to go to their bedroom or another area specifically identified for this purposes.

Staff should create time for the person to think, including giving them a quiet place to go, and prompts which aid contemplation, e.g.

- staff establishing rapport and trust by acknowledging the feelings of the service user through reflective listening; the feelings that led the individual to use challenging behaviour;
- the service user is given space to explore events that precipitated the behaviour;
- staff to commend the service user through praise for their effort to calm themselves down, a service user might expect to be criticised or blamed for their behaviour, whatever, their expectations staff should affirm their courage by saying something like 'I'm impressed you calmed yourself quickly'; praising the service user's demonstration of responsibility increases their confidence

Where personal space has been identified as physical intervention support strategy, it should be clearly written down into the individual's physical intervention policy along with strict guidelines as to what staff support of the individual needs during this time. If the individual chooses to go to their bedroom, staff must always be in close proximity of the room/area.

11.16 Recording an incident

When recording an incident it is essential to use the reflective practice model. Experience in itself does not always result in professional development; some people do not learn from experience and repeat the same mistakes

11.16.1 What is reflective practice?

Reflective practice is a way of thinking which adds value to experience and enables people to benefit from it.

> Reflective practice is something more than thoughtful practice. It is that form of practice that seeks to problematise many situations of professional performance so that they can become potential learning situations and so the practitioners can continue to learn, grow and develop in and through practice. (Jarvis, 1992: 180).

11.16.2 Why do we reflect?

- We reflect in order to engage in personal and self-development and in order to make decisions or resolve uncertainty.
- Simply having and experiencing is not sufficient. Reflection upon this experience is needed in order to learn from it; without reflection, experiences are often quickly forgotten and therefore the opportunity for development is lost.
- The feelings and thoughts developed through reflection are what generate concepts and it is through these concepts that we learn and accordingly adapt our attitudes, beliefs and actions. (Gibbs, 1988)

11.16.3 When do we reflect?

We reflect:

- when something went really well;
- during a crisis/incident;
- during an uncomfortable situation;
- during a situation where what usually works is not working;
- on an occasion when a usual explanation did not suffice, prompting the need for a new explanation.

11.16.4 Stages in reflective practice

By thinking through incidents in a structured way, accidental, informal and everyday practice can be converted into effective learning opportunities. There are six stages involved when recording an incident using reflective practice. These stages are:

1. Describe the event in detail
2. Describe your feelings
3. Evaluation
4. Analysis
5. Conclusion
6. Action plan

Stage 1: Description of the event

Describe in details the event you are reflecting on:

- Where were you?
- Who else was there?
- Why were you there?
- What were you doing?
- What were the other people doing?
- What was the context of the event?
- What happened?
- What was your part in this?

- What parts did the other people play?
- What was the result?

Stage 2: Describe your feelings

Recalling and exploring your feelings after an event enables you to explore the links between feelings and actions. It allows you to explore and identify the meaning behind your 'gut instinct':

- How were you feeling when the event started?
- What were you thinking at that time?
- What were you thinking about when it happened?
- How did it make you feel then?
- What did other people's actions/words make you think?
- What did these make you feel?
- How did you feel about the outcome of the event?
- What do you think about it now?
- What were the emotions that you have gone through from the start to the finish of the event?
- Which of these is more significant or important to you?

Stage 3: Evaluation

When people evaluate situations they are comparing outcomes to a level of expected standards. By doing this, they are able to reach a judgment about what happened.

- What was good about the event?
- What was not good about the event?
- Why was it important?

Stage 4: Analysis

Analysing an event allows people to break down the events into components parts so they can be explored separately. At this point you will need to ask more detailed questions about the answers to the last stage (Evaluation stage):

- What went well?
- What did you do well?
- What did others do well?
- What went wrong?
- What caught you by surprise?
- In what ways did your action or lack of actions contribute to this?
- In what ways did others actions or lack of actions contribute to this?
- Why might these things have happened?

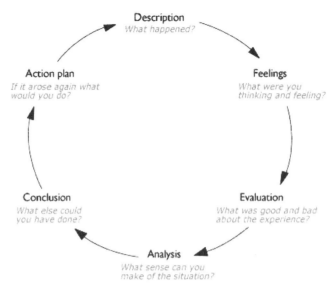

Figure 11.1 The reflective cycle (Gibbs, 1988).

Stage 5: Conclusion

It is at this stage that you will likely develop insight into your own and other people's behaviour in terms of how they contributed to the outcome of event. Keep in mind that the purpose of reflection is to learn from an experience. Without detailed analysis and honest exploration that occurs during all the previous stages, it is not likely that all aspects of the event will be taken into account and thus a valuable chance for learning can be lost. During this stage you should ask yourself:

* What can be done differently next time?

Stage 6: Action plan

At this stage you should think yourself forward into encountering the event again and plan what you would do. Ask yourself:

* Would you act differently?
* Would you be likely to do the same?

11.17 Learning outcomes

* To demonstrate an understanding of the application of risk management interventions and the requirements for the effective assessment of dangerousness with reference to prevention planning;
* To demonstrate an understanding of restraint-related risks, as outlined in the Bennett Inquiry and NICE guidelines with a view to incorporating risk reduction strategies into practice.
* To demonstrate an understanding of the need for and scope of post-incident review procedures and of how to identify strategies and interventions for future prevention.

226

- To identify spheres of influence in relation to the individual, team and organisational change required to achieve a reduction in aggression and violence.

11.18 Framework for reflective practice

- ➢ *Knowledge:* What have you learnt from reading this chapter?
- ➢ *Skills:* What do you know, or can do differently now, that you did not/could not do before reading this chapter?
- ➢ *Practices:* How can you perform a task now better than before?

11.19 References

Bryan, F., Allan, T., Russell, L. (2000) The move from a long-stay learning disabilities hospital to community homes: A comparison of clients' nutritional status, *Journal of Human Nutrition and Dietetics* **13**(4): 265–70.

Clements, C. and Martin, N. (2002) *Assessing Behaviours Regarded as Problematic for People with Developmental Disabilities*. London: Jessica Kingsley.

Clements, J. (2005) *People with Autism Behaving Badly: Helping People with ASD Move On from Behavioural and Emotional Challenges*. London: Jessica Kingsley.

Crisis Prevention Institute (2002) Seven Principles for Effective Verbal Intervention. Crisis Prevention Institute, Inc. http://www.crisisprevention.com

David, A. (ed.) (2003) *Ethical Approaches to Physical Interventions: Responding to Challenging Behaviour in People with Intellectual Disabilities*. London: British Institute of Learning Disabilities.

Department for Education and Skills (2002) Guidance on the use of restrictive physical interventions for Pupils with Severe Behavioural Difficulties. Nottingham: DIES Publications.

Department of Health (2002) *Guidance for Restrictive Physical Intervention*. London: DoH.

Department of Health & Welsh Office (1999) *The Mental Health Act Code of Practice*. London: DoH.

Dilworth, K. (2000) *Literature Review (Teenage Pregnancy)*. Canadian Institute of Child Health. (http://www.phac-aspc.gc.ca/dca- dea /publications/reduce_teen_pregnancy_section_2_e.html).

Emerson, E. (1995) *Challenging Behaviour: Analysis and Intervention in People with Learning Disabilities*. Cambridge: Cambridge University Press.

Emerson, E. (2001) *Challenging Behaviour: Analysis and Intervention in People with Learning Disabilities*, 2nd edn. Cambridge: Cambridge University Press.

Gibbs, G (1988) *Learning by Doing: A guide to teaching and learning methods*. Oxford: Further Education Unit. Oxford Polytechnic: Oxford.

Gray, C. and McAndrew, S. (2001) *My Social Stories Book*. London: Jessica Kingsley Publishers.

Greene, R.W. (2005) *The Explosive Child*. New York: HarperCollins .

Greene, R.W. and Ablon, J.S. (2005) *Treating Explosive Kids: The Collaborative Problem Solving Approach*. New York: Guilford.

Hardy, S. and Joyce, T. (2011) *Challenging Behaviour: A Handbook: Practical Resource Addressing Ways of Providing Positive Behavioural Support to People with Learning Disabilities Whose Behaviour is Described as Challenging*. Brighton: Pavilion Publishing Ltd.

Harris, J., Allen, D., Cornick, M., Jefferson, A., et al. (1996) *Physical Interventions. A Policy Framework*. British Institute of Learning Disabilities.

Hieneman, M. and Dunlap, G. (1999) Issues and challenges in implementing community-based behavioral support for two boys with severe disabilities. In J.R. Scotti and L.H. Meyer (eds), *Behavioral Intervention: Principles, Models, and Practices*, Baltimore: Paul H. Brookes, pp. 363–84.

Jarvis, P. (1992) Reflective practice and nursing. *Nurse Education Today* **12**: 174–81.

Lennox, N. and Diggens, J. (2005) *Management Guidelines for People with Developmental and Intellectual Disabilities*. Melbourne: Therapeutic Guidelines Ltd.

Linsley P. (2006) *Violence and Aggression in the Work Place: A Practical Guide for All Health Care Staff.* Oxford: Radcliffe Publishing.

Rippon, T.J. (2000) Aggression and violence in health care professions, *Journal of Advanced Nursing* **31**(2): 452–60.

Royal College of Psychiatrists, British Psychological Society & Royal College of Speech and Language Therapists (2007) *Challenging Behaviour: A Unified Approach.* London: RCP, BPS and RCSLT.

Shore, S.M. and Rastelli, L.G. (2006) *Understanding Autism for Dummies.* Chichester: John Wiley & Sons, Ltd.

11.20 Induction workbook

1. Why is it important to be aware that a service user may have unpredictable moods and behaviour?

2. What are the likely dangers to be created by these unpredictable moods and behaviour?

3. Explain why behaviour may be an important form of communication for some people with learning disabilities.

4. Give five examples of how behaviour may be a way of communicating feelings, choices, needs and views.

5. Outline the method used in your organization to manage challenging behaviour?

6. What strategies are used to motivate and control challenging behaviour in a care setting?

PART IV

MAINTAINING SAFETY AT WORK

12   Health and Safety

AIMS

- To gain an understanding of the importance of health and safety at work
- To understand how hazards are identified
- To understand risks assessment and the principles of control measures
- To develop a culture of safety consciousness at the workplace
- To recognise legal aspects of health and safety
- To identify the types of hazards at workplace and measures to control them
- To become risk-conscious at all times

12.1   Introduction: what is health and safety at work?

Health and safety at work is a government regulation that is used to protect the employee in a working environment. An employee has to enjoy the following rights; to have any risks to their health and safety properly controlled, to be provided, free of charge, with any personal protective and safety equipment

12.2   Brief guide to health and safety law: key points

Your health, safety and welfare at work are protected by law. Your employer has a duty to protect and keep you informed about health and safety at your workplace. You, as an employee, have a responsibility to look after yourself and others.

    Your employer has a duty under the Health and Safety at Work Act 1974 and the Management of Health and Safety at Work Regulations of 1999 (as amended) and related legislation including the Environmental Protection Act 1990 and the Fire Precautions Act 1971, to ensure, so far as is reasonably practical, your health, safety and welfare at work.

12.2.1   Employers' responsibilities

- Provide health and safe systems of work, including a safe working environment, and premises with adequate amenities.
- Provide safe access and exit to and from the workplace.
- Ensure that staff have appropriate training, instructions and supervision.
- Supply adequate information to employees so that they can ensure their own health and safety at work, and that of the people they work with.
- Have a written health and safety policy.
- Provide safe plants, machinery, equipment and appliances, and safe methods of handling, storing and transporting materials.
- Avoid hazardous manual handling operations, and where they cannot be avoided, reduce the risk of injury.
- Provide health surveillance as appropriate like CCTV to reduce the risk of damage, violence and disruption in the service.
- Ensure that appropriate safety signs are provided and maintained, e.g. exit signs on doors.

- Report certain injuries, diseases and dangerous occurrences to the appropriate health and safety enforcing authority.
- Set up emergency procedures like fire evacuations.

Additional requirements include:

- Taking reasonable care to ensure the safety of visitors to properties, including contractors working on-site, and telling them about any known hazards.
- To make sure that premises are free from defects.

12.2.2 Employees' responsibilities

As an employee you have legal duties and obligations to comply with individual duties under Section 7 of Health and Safety at Work Act 1974, regulation 14 of the Management of Health and Safety at Work regulations 1999. Employees have a duty to:

- take reasonable care of themselves and anyone else who might be affected by what they do at work or do not do;
- co-operate with the employer on health and safety matters;
- use correctly work items provided by the employer, including:
  o personal protective equipment, in accordance with training or instructions;
  o not interfering with or misuse anything provided for their health, safety or welfare at work.

12.2.3 Working practices

- Employees must not operate any item of equipment unless they have been trained and/or authorised to do so.
- Employees must report to management or senior members of staff immediately any faulty defects or malfunction on any item of equipment, fixture or fitting which could cause danger to anyone.
- Employees must not carry out any repairs or maintenance work of any description unless authorised to do so.
- Employees must use all liquid substances, detergents etc., in accordance with written instructions and never transfer detergent/liquid substances in a container other than its original container.
- Employees must dress in a manner appropriate to the task they will be expected to undertake.

12.2.4 Fire precautions

- Employees must make themselves aware of the location of all fire escape routes from the premises.
- Employees must not obstruct or cause obstruction to any fire escape routes.
- Employees will be expected to undertake training on the actions to be taken in the event of a fire emergency and to know what actions they will be expected to take.
- Employees must consider the safety of those in their care in all instances of a fire emergency and understand the evacuation procedures.
- Employees must be aware of the homes/project/schemes' individual fire risk assessment.

12.2.5 Working conditions/environment

- Employees must make proper use of all facilities provided not only for the safety of themselves, but of those in their care
- All employees must dispose of all rubbish or infected materials and foods wastes in the manner prescribed and using the disposal methods and equipment provided. For example:
  o sharps in the yellow sharps container provided; this will include needles and syringes;
  o used bandages and dressing and soiled pads in a yellow plastic bag with plastic fasteners for disposal;
  o soiled clothing in the red bags before putting them in the washing machine.
- All employees must assist in keeping stairways, passageways and work areas clear and in neat and tidy condition.
- All employees must clear up all spillages promptly and advise others that they have to cross recently 'mopped' slippery areas by displaying safety warning triangles.

12.2.6 Accidents/illnesses

- Employees must notify the management or a manager/team leader of any incident, which causes injury/near miss or damage to property.
- Employees must seek medical attention or advice for any injury or illness that they may be suffering from, any treatment, no matter how slight, should be recorded in the accident book and reported to the line manager.

12.2.7 Legislation and regulations on health and safety (HSE)

The following legislation and regulations promote awareness and understanding of health and safety throughout the workforce:

- Health and Safety at Work etc. Act 1974
- The Management of Health and Safety at Work Regulations of 1999

Related legislation includes:

- Environmental Protection Act 1990
- Fire Precautions Act 1971
- Reporting of Injuries, Diseases and Dangerous Occurrences Regulations 1995 (RIDDOR)
- Health and Safety Information for Employees Regulations 1989
- Personal Protective Equipment Regulations 1992
- Provision and Use of Work Equipment Regulations 1998
- Workplace (Health, Safety, and Welfare) Regulations 1992
- Lifting Operations and Lifting Equipment Regulations 1998

12.2.8 National health and safety guidelines in the workplace

- All staff and service users are obligated where appropriate to report hazards and to manage them in the first instance.
- All activities which are undertaken by staff have been risk assessed and management controls have been devised to manage them and all those taking part sign the risk assessment.

- Staff who are working alone either in a project or in a client's home must follow the policies and procedures which detail what actions they should take to manage risks which may arise when lone working.
- To ensure a good standard of health and safety, and to maintain a good state of repairs:
  o staff should carry out basic building checks and report any building defects;
  o fire checks on a weekly basis testing the fire alarms and smoke detectors to ensure they are in good working order.
- Every service should possess first-aid kits to manage minor injuries of self-harm which the clients/service users may present.

12.3 How to involve service users/clients in national health and safety policy

When making decisions on risks and how to manage them, it must be recognised that intervention by staff or others can increase risks as well as decrease them. The interaction between service users and staff are crucial to the assessment and management of risk. Good relationships make assessment easier and are more accurate and may reduce risk. Risks may be increased if relationships are poor.

- Service users should be encouraged where appropriate to address their concerns about facilities they have access to in their homes/care setting during link work or key working sessions.
- As participants in the management of health and safety, service users are expected to participate in the local health and safety policy based on the four concepts of:
  o risk identification;
  o risk reporting;
  o risk assessment;
  o risk management.
- As participants in activities that carry risk, service users should, where appropriate, be invited to sign and contribute to risk assessment.
- Service users should be encouraged to report any problems around their homes/projects and living environment during in-house or team meetings or any concerns which the management of the organisation seek to address.

12.4 Four concepts in local health and safety implementation

12.4.1 Risk identification

The risks service users face or present should be routinely assessed and kept under review as part of the referral, assessment and support planning process. When identifying risks, the assessment and management should as far as possible be based on objective information. In summary:

- Risk identification should be carried out by staff with new service user moving into a residential home/care setting/project and recorded.
- Staff and service users should be vigilant in their observation of their living/working environment and bring any potential risks or hazards to the attention of the management.
- Periodic checks should be carried out around buildings, at least once a week; fire checks and monthly thorough defects action checks should be completed as outlined in the maintenance policy to ensure good standards of health and safety.

- Regular building and security checks should be performed in order to increase the likelihood of noticing any risks or health and safety hazards.
- New referrals should be discussed in team meetings in order to maximise the opportunity to identify risks with individual service user.

12.4.2 Risk reporting

- Service users where appropriate, should be expected to report any hazards that they may notice to members of staff.
- Staff should highlight hazards and risks during building checks or fire checks and report them to the management or log them with the maintenance team.
- If serious risks or health and safety violations occur, e.g. in case of a fire or flooding, the incident should be reported in accordance with the major incident procedure.

12.4.3 Risk assessment

A risk assessment is an analysis of hazards in the work/living place. Assessments ensure that safe procedures happen. Procedures state: who does what, when and how?

- Risk assessments should be carried out and written about all risks which are noticed, with regard to the service, be it building or service users based.
- In order for all risk assessments to be in line with Health and Safety Regulations, they should be viewed and approved by the line/project/home managers.
- All risk assessments should be reviewed and updated regularly (at least every six months depending on the nature of the risk) and current and new control measures should be implemented if it is felt necessary at that time.
- Risk assessments should be passed to the service/line/home manager for auditing purposes and to ensure that all national and local health and safety guidelines have been adhered to.

12.4.4 Risk management

- Risk assessment should be carried out when a risk has been noticed. Once a risk assessment has been performed, all staff members should read and sign that risk assessment, and implement all procedures as indicated to minimise the risk or eliminate it.
- Any risk brought to the attention of the management should be reviewed regularly to ensure that all measures possible are being taken to minimise the risk of potential harm.
- If it is felt the risk needs immediate attention, then all necessary measures should be taken or contact the relevant agencies or the police to immediately deal with the risk as soon as possible.

12.5 Maintenance policy

Information regarding this policy for buildings maintenance is maintained by the Organisations (Employers) in Maintenance Manual which is designed to ensure that buildings meet all legal obligations as detailed in the following legal regulations:

- Health and Safety at Work Act 1974
- Occupiers Liability Act 1957

- Management of Health and Safety at Work Regulations 1992
- The Workplace (Health, Safety and Welfare) Regulations 1992
- Control of Substances Hazardous to Health (COSHH) 1988
- Defective Premises Act 1972
- Gas (Installation and Use) 1998
- Furniture and Furnishing (Fire Safety) Regulations 1988
- Food Safety Act 1990
- Food Hygiene (General) Regulations (as Amended) 1970
- Registered Care Homes Act 1984
- Fire Precautions (Workplace) 1997
- Control of Asbestos at Work 1987

12.6   Learning outcomes

- To understand the importance of acting in ways that are consistent with legislation, policies and procedures for maintaining own and others' health and safety.
- To know how to identify and report any issues at work that may put health and safety at risk.
- To be able to identify and assess the potential risks involved in work activities and processes for self and others.
- To understand individual responsibilities in reporting incidents and know details of the policies and processes in place for reporting such incidents.
- To understand the need to co-operate with employer on health and safety matters and correctly use work items provided by their employer, including personal protective equipment, and moving and handling equipment in accordance with training or instructions.
- To understand that individuals must not misuse anything provided for their and others' health, safety or welfare.

12.7   Framework for reflective practice

➢ *Knowledge:*   What have you learnt from reading this chapter?
➢ *Skills:*   What do you know, or can do differently now, that you did not/could not do before reading this chapter?
➢ *Practices:*   How can you perform a task now better than before?

12.8   References

Health and Safety (Training for Employment) Regulations 1990.

Health and Safety at Work Act etc. 1974.

HM Government – Fire Safety Risk Assessment: 'Means of Escape for Disabled People'.

HSE (1974) Health and Safety at Work etc. Act 1974 – available at
http://www.hse.gov.uk/legislation/hswa.htm

HSE (1999) Management of Health and Safety at Work Regulations 1999.
http://www.hse.gov.uk/pubns/hsc13.pdf

HSE (1999) Management of Health & Safety at Work Regulations, 1999. Approved Code of Practice & Guidance (L21).

HSE (2011) Five Steps to Risk Assessment (available at www.hse.gov.uk/pubns/indg163.pdf

Management of Health and Safety at Work and Fire Precautions (Workplace) (Amendment) Regulations 2003

Safety Representatives and Safety Committees Regulations 1977.

12.9 Induction workbook

1. Give a brief summary of the Health and Safety Policy.
   _____
   _____

2. How would you involve service users in your organisation in participating in health and safety?
   _____
   _____

3. Do service users have any responsibilities in terms of health and safety?
   _____
   _____

4. What legislations and regulations promote awareness and understanding of health and safety throughout the workforce?
   _____
   _____

5. Outline the national health and safety guidelines in the workplace.
   _____
   _____

6. What are the four concepts in local health and safety implementation?
   _____
   _____

7. What is risk assessment and risk management? How are they used to promote health and safety at work?
   _____
   _____

13 Administration, Documentation and Storage of Medication

AIMS

- To ensure that all staff are competent and confident to perform all duties relating to medication in a safe and responsible manner
- To provide an introduction to medication within a care setting
- To provide the terms and procedure used when dispensing medication to the service user
- To provide the terms and procedures of storing and documenting medication

13.1 Introduction to administration of medication

As you develop new skills, you are expected to apply them in a safe manner.

- This includes ensuring that you work within the approved guidelines, and do not knowingly take action that is known to be detrimental to the service user.
- There are times when you will need advice from other professionals. Their decisions will be based on a broader, in-depth knowledge greater than your own. However, you must never take action suggested by others that you know to be harmful to the service user.
- Following orders is not an excuse for doing something you know to be wrong.

13.2 Accountability and responsibility

Responsibility and accountability are often used interchangeably but they are different.

- If you are held responsible, you are expected to carry out the activity or duties to the best of your ability.
- If you are held accountable you are obliged to account for your actions to someone who has the right to ask. This means giving an explanation.
- However, you can be held responsible without being accountable, but not vice versa.
- With both accountability and responsibility, you are obliged to keep your knowledge and skills up-to-date.

As a social care worker administering medicines, you need to be clear as to your responsibilities and accountability.

13.2.1 Who are you accountable to and how?

- You are accountable to the organisation, through your terms and conditions of employment, which means you are expected to follow the organisation's policies and procedures which are contained within the manual for reference, all of which are written to safeguard the service user, the organisation and you. Failure to adhere to the policies and procedures can result in action being taken against you.

- Whilst you are accountable to the organisation, you must never follow their orders unquestionably, as you are also accountable to others.
- Accountability and responsibility is not just about doing something right. You are also at risk if you are aware of something happening which you know to be wrong and you take no action.

13.3   Legislation requirements governing the management of medicines

There are two main statutes of law called 'Acts' from which regulations and orders arise that contribute to the regulations of medication within a care setting:

- The Medicines Act 1968
- The Misuse of Drugs Act 1971

The Medicines Act (1968) and the Misuse of Drugs Act (1971) dictates how medicines are managed and they must be complied with.

- Under the Medicines 1968 Act, a pharmacist must supervise the supply of medicines, and check that prescriptions are dispensed by an order from an authorised prescriber.
- The Misuse of Drugs 1971 Act imposes additional controls on medicines that are potentially addictive and are designated as 'dangerous' or otherwise harmful.
- These 'prescriptions only medicines' are called Controlled Drugs (CDs) and there are additional legal requirements laid down as to their storage, prescribing and use.
- The special way that these drugs are managed may be extended to include other medicines.

13.4   Drug classes

All drugs are given legal category to control how they are supplied to the public. The following abbreviations may be found on the packaging:

- POM   Prescription Only Medication
- P   Pharmacy Medicines: these medicines may only be sold in the pharmacy and the pharmacist must supervise the sale
- GSL   General Sales List: these medicines may only be sold in other stores such as supermarkets. Also known as household medicine

Occasionally you may come across other abbreviations either on the prescription or on the packaging. These are abbreviations for Latin words:

- TD   Twice Daily
- TDS   Three Times Daily
- QDS   Four Times Daily
- STAT   Immediately
- NOCTE Night

- MAINE   Morning
- PRN   As and when required

13.5   Medication policy and procedure

This guideline should be read with a MAR sheet. See Figure 13.1.

- Many of the service users require regular medication to maintain their physical and/or mental health. As they find it difficult to manage safely, in most cases they will rely on you to ensure they are given the correct dose at the appropriate time.
- These guidelines will help you carry out this task safely and efficiently.
- Medications used in residential/care settings can be harmful/hazardous therefore, please ensure that safe practice is observed.

13.5.1   Medication Administration Record (MAR) sheet

MAR sheets stands for Medication Administration Record sheets.

- These sheets are the principal records kept at all residential homes. They detail:

    o   the name of the service user;
    o   the drugs supplied to each service user;
    o   in what quantity;
    o   what time and by whom.

- They also include carbonated orders and checking sheets.
- MAR sheets come from the designated pharmacy like Boots pharmacy and are part of the Boots medication service used by the company.
- The left-hand box of the MAR sheets shows the chemical name of the medication, the trade name if any, and the strength (in milligrams) of each tablet.
- For liquid medication the strength is usually shown in weight of the active ingredient in a particular volume. For example, 25 mg/5 ml indicates that every 5 ml contains 25 mg of the drug.
- The next box indicates how many tablets, or what volume of liquid should be given, and at what time. Note that the dose may vary at different times of the day.
- The following series of boxes are for staff members responsible for giving out the medication to confirm that it has been done.
- There is one column for each day of the month. This should be initialled/signed by staff who administer the medication only after the service user has swallowed medication.
- The MAR sheet can be useful tool for the care provider to use to keep track of medicines that are not ordered every month but only taken occasionally.
- Where for any reason the dose is not given, the following letters should be entered in the box in place of a signature.

A refused
B nausea/vomit
C hospitalised
D social leave
E refused & destroyed
F other
G see note overleaf

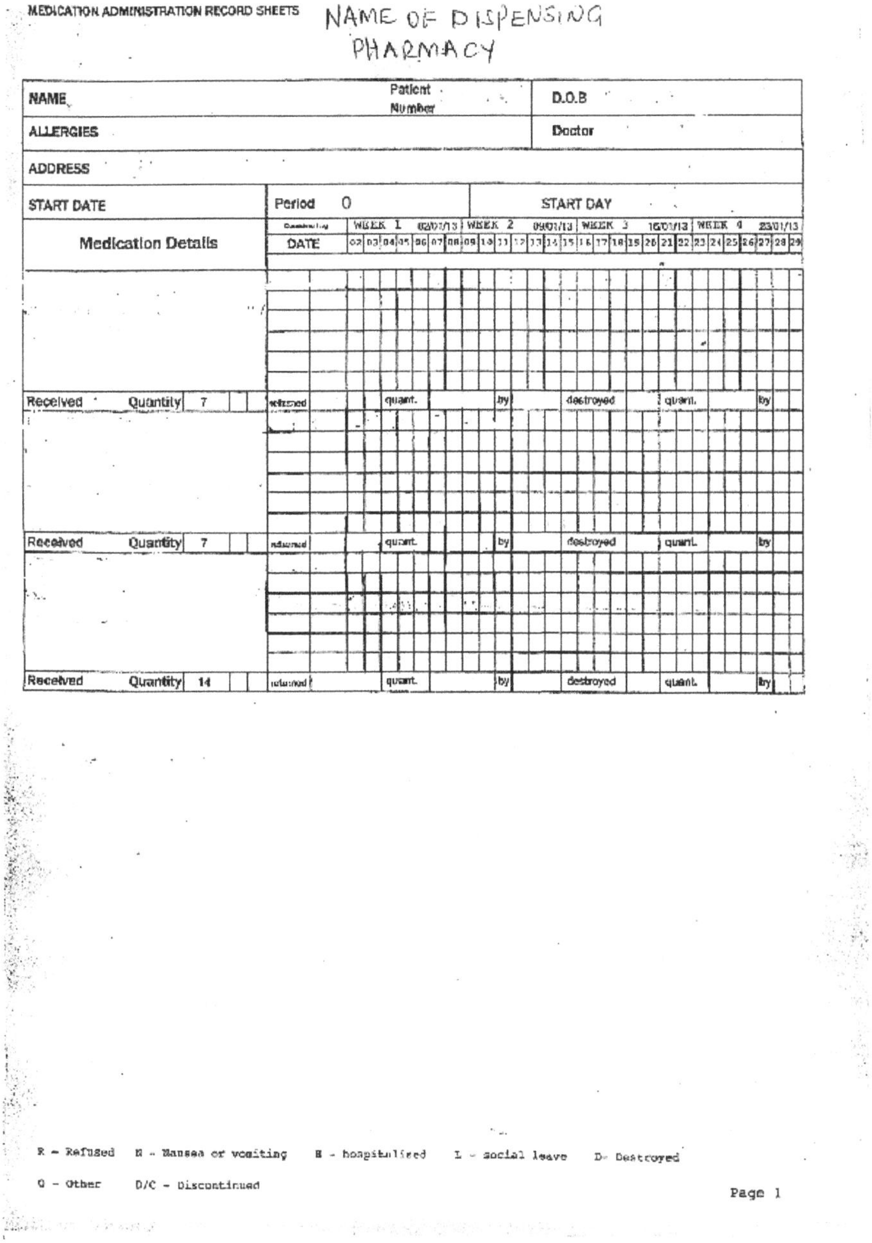
MEDICATION ADMINISTRATION RECORD SHEETS
NAME OF DISPENSING PHARMACY
NAME
Patient Number
D.O.B
ALLERGIES
Doctor
ADDRESS
START DATE
Period 0
START DAY
Medication Details
WEEK 1 02/01/13
WEEK 2 09/01/13
WEEK 3 16/01/13
WEEK 4 23/01/13
DATE 02 03 04 05 06 07 08 09 10 11 12 13 14 15 16 17 18 19 20 21 22 23 24 25 26 27 28 29
Received Quantity 7 returned quant. by destroyed quant. by
Received Quantity 7 returned quant. by destroyed quant. by
Received Quantity 14 returned quant. by destroyed quant. by
R – Refused N – Nausea or vomiting H – hospitalised L – social leave D– Destroyed
O – Other D/C – Discontinued
Page 1

Figure 13.1 MAR sheet.

13.5.2 Procedures for the administration of medication

In order to reduce the potential for errors the following procedure should be adhered to when administering medication.

- Prepare the work area and any equipment necessary, ensuring plentiful supply of clean and dry medication pots, beakers, large jug of water, pens, medication file (MAR sheet), medication cabinet keys, protective gloves and then wash your hands.
- Open the medication folder of the first service user and using the appropriate blister pack holder for the time of day (am, noon, 6 pm and 10 pm) begin the process of popping tablets from the blister pack into the pot in the following manner:
- Read the first item on the MAR sheet; check the relevant blister pack to ensure the label on the pack is the same as the medication listed on the MAR sheet and pop into the medication pot. Staff should initial relevant box to say medication has been dispensed. Repeat until all medication in tablet form for the one service user, for the time of the day is dispensed and signed for.
- Do not leave the signing until you have finished each person. Ensure you sign every item each time. This will also assist if you need to stop dispensing, as you will always know where you have to go.
- It is important to note that some medication is not blister packed and remains in its original packaging in the medication cabinet. These will have reminder cards on the folder and will be dispensed the same way i.e. by checking that the label on the packaging is the same as that on the MAR sheet and dispense into a medication pot.
- Once the required number of tablets have been removed from the non-blister pack, the remainder of that medication should be returned to the medication cabinet.
- Liquid medication should be dispensed into separate pot dry from dry medication unless there are specific instructions from the pharmacist to do otherwise.
- Where medication needs to be crushed and mixed with liquid, this should be checked by staff against the MAR sheet and then administered to the relevant service user with at least half a beaker of water. Service users should be encouraged to come to the office or delegated medication area where the medication is stored and take their medication from there. Only the service user receiving his/her medication at that time should be in the room.
- When you have observed the medication that has been administered being swallowed with the aid of water from the beaker, initial or sign to show evidence medication has been dispensed and administered. For controlled drugs such as Temazapam, the controlled drug book also needs completing each time the medication is given, remembering to record the number of tablets remaining
- All the above stages need repeating until all the medication has been dispensed, administered and recorded appropriately.

Note: some service users may require medication that is not taken orally, for example inhalers, creams or eye drops and it may be more appropriate for these to be administered by the member of staff providing that service user with personal care. In this instance, the MAR sheet recording and signing must be carried out as detailed above.

13.5.3 Medication administration

When administering medication, staff should know the therapeutic use of the medication administered, its normal dose, side effects, precautions and contra-indications of each drug. Follow this procedure:

- Select the service user's MAR sheet.
- Make sure the prescribed dose has not already been administered and note any changes in treatment (increase or decrease in dosage).
- Check that the prescription or the label on the medication is clear and unambiguous and relates to the service user in person.
- Check the identity of the service user (against the photograph on the medication folder).
- Administer the medication.
- Record on the MAR sheet immediately after the medicine has been taken.
- Record if the medicine is not taken and state the reason on the MAR sheet.
- Where medicine is taken from the container and not taken by the service user, it should be stored in an envelope marked contaminated and returned to the dispensing chemist. It should never be replaced back in the container.
- Where the service user refuses to take their medicines, this should be reported to a senior member of staff or the manager who will then decide on what action to take or call NHS direct for advice. However, this is dependent on the nature of drugs prescribed.

13.5.4 Routes of administration

The route of medicines means the way in which medicines are taken or administered. Staff should never administer medicine, but support service users to self-administer; the only exception to this is following prolonged seizures, only when directed by an individual care plan, and administered by a fully trained staff.

- intra-aural – into the ears;
- inhalation – by nose or mouth into the lungs;
- intra-ocular – into the eyes;
- oral – by mouth;
- intramuscular – drug injected into the large muscle in the arm, leg or buttocks;
- intravenous – injected directly into a vein or cannula;
- rectal – introduced into the rectum through the anus;
- sublingual – under the tongue;
- topical – applied to the outer surface of the body, e.g. skin.

13.5.5 Procedure for the use of non-prescribed medication

- It is important to remember that you are not employed as a medical practitioner and should not therefore make decisions about medication people you are supporting require, without taking advice from suitably qualified medical practitioner.
- All prescribed medication must be given exactly as instructed, unless advice has been sought from the person who prescribed it to adjust the time/dose as appropriate.

- Non-prescribed medication, such as simple cough linctus, should rarely be necessary as on most occasions someone who is unwell enough to need medication should be supported to see their GP.
- There are occasions when this is not necessary – for example with an occasional headache; on these occasions an over-the-counter remedy may be appropriate. However, medical advice should still be sought.

This is to ensure that the proposed remedy:

- would not adversely affect prescribed medication already being taken;
- is appropriate for that particular individual and their medical history;
- is an appropriate treatment for the ailment causing discomfort.

All medication will be booked in using the procedure in place even if that medication is a non-prescribed remedy.

- All medication should be administered in accordance with the procedure and its use recorded in the same way regardless of how it was obtained.
- Service users should never share medication. A supply of any medication needed for an individual will be purchased on his/her behalf when necessary and be disposed at the end of its shelf life.

13.5.6 As required ('PRN') medication

- 'As required' medication is prescribed by a GP or hospital to treat various symptoms occurring on an irregular basis.
- These symptoms may include anxiety, maniac depression, tremors, and constipation among many others.
- It is therefore important that the prescribed medication is offered at the appropriate time for each individual.
- Suggestions as to when it might be given should be supported by a care plan for staff to follow.

While the circumstances leading to the administration of many PRN drugs may be stressful to the service user and staff, it is important to bear in mind the following points:

1. Taking the medication is voluntary on the part of the service user, and they must give an informed consent before taking it (that means they must be made aware of the effect of the medication and why they are being asked to take it) e.g. 'You seem rather upset at the moment, these tablets will make you feel calmer.' Or something similar that would be appropriate way of raising the matter with the service user
2. All drugs are dangerous if taken in overdose, in which case some may be fatal. They may have side effects requiring other medication at a later stage. It is essential, therefore, that any administration of these drugs is fully recorded on the medication sheet for the service user concerned. This should show:

- time of administration;
- dose given;
- initials of the staff giving the medication.

3. After a service user has taken any psychotropic (e.g. sedative or tranquillising) drugs their condition should be monitored at least half hourly, and if any symptoms, e.g. breathing, colour, temperature, gives cause for concern the GP and the on-call manager should be informed immediately or call the paramedics depending on your assessment of the individual.

4. No orally administered drug is a 'magic wand' and may take several hours to be absorbed into the system and give any noticeable effect.

5. 'Household medicines': These include the following commercially available preparations: Aspirin, Paracetamol, commercial cough mixtures, and indigestion remedies. Although not strictly 'as required', the administration of these remedies must be ordered in the same way as that of any other medication, and the manufacturers stated dose strictly adhered to.

Note: Never be afraid to consult a shift leader or on-call manager (in case of lone working) if you are in any way concerned, even in cases where a referral is not mandatory.

13.5.7   Use of PRN medication

Service users who are prescribed PRN medication may be given the appropriate doses without having to contact a doctor beforehand. However, it is important to contact the on-call manager, and if there is any doubt about when to give PRN, refer to the care plan in place and consult a senior member of staff

13.6   General information on medication

- Any increase or decrease in dosage must be authorised by a doctor. If this is done over the telephone, record the change and the name of the doctor in the service user's daily diary and notify all staff through the communication book.
- No one can be given medication prescribed for another service user except with the express authorisation of a doctor.
- Information on different medicines and their side effects can be found in the British National Formulary (BNF), a copy of which is kept in the offices of all care settings.
- If in doubt: ask, don't guess.

13.6.1   Rectal medication

Only staff that have been given formal instructions and training and deemed competent by the trainer may administer rectal medication.

13.6.2   How medication arrives in the home/project

Medication is normally given to service users' homes in four different forms:

1. *Monitored Dosage System (MDS) (otherwise called a blister pack)*

   - Here the pharmacy put the tablets and capsules into plastic bubbles that are sealed onto a card.
   - Each blister pack usually contains 28 days' supply of medication for a particular time of day.
   - The medication is released from the pack by pushing the plastic bubble, which in turn pushes the tablet/capsule through the metal foil at the back of the card.

   A colour system is used with the blister packs:

   - pink for morning
   - yellow for lunchtime
   - orange for evening
   - blue for night medication
   - white blister packs – a course of antibiotics or medication when required.

2. *Sealed packs*

These are similar to the monitored dosage system but each pack contains only one tablet/capsule.

3. *Bottles for tablets/capsules*

These are usually brown glass bottles with screw caps.

4. *Bottles for liquids*

These are usually brown glass bottles with screw caps

13.6.3 Labelling of medication

All four types will be clearly labelled with the name of the service user, the medication and dose, when and how to administer.

13.6.4 Storage of medication

   - The organisation is ultimately responsible for the safe storage and security of medicines. The project/home manager has 24-hour responsibility. This means that they are responsible for ensuring that policies and procedures are adhered to, even in their absence. The shift leader on duty is responsible during their shift for the storage and security of medicines.
   - The cupboard where the medication is stored must be kept locked at all times and the keys must be kept with the shift leader on duty at all times or, in case of lone working, the staff on duty must adhere to the same rules.
   - Items should be stored in designated clean areas and arranged tidily in the order that they were received. This means: a system of stock rotation can be operated, there is no accumulation of 'old' stock and items are used before their expiry date.

- The temperature of the environment may affect a drug's suitability (performance) so no medicinal preparation should be stored where it may be subjected to a wide variation in temperature.

13.6.5 Storage of controlled drugs

- Controlled drugs (CDs) are stored in a secure, usually metal, cupboard that is used exclusively for the storage of CDs and those drugs that are managed in the same way.
- The cupboard which is often contained within a second cupboard is kept locked and access is restricted.
- The quantity and supply of these drugs is recorded in a controlled drug register. This book is to be kept near the cupboard where the CD are stored at all times and entries in it should be made, and checked by two staff, one of whom should be the shift leader.

13.6.6 The title of a medicine and its name

- Each medicine has two names, a generic (non-proprietary), titles and a brand name.
- The generic title is based on the medicine's main ingredients.
- The brand name is the name which the manufacturer markets the drug by.

For example: carbomazapine is the generic name for Tegretol. Tegretol is the brand name which is used to regulate epilepsy and mood swings; or the antipsychotic brand drug called Clopixol has a generic name of zuclopenthixol.

13.6.7 Possible errors that can be made when administering medication

- Not administering medication.
- Not administering enough medication.
- Administering too much medication.
- Administering wrong medication.
- Administering medication to the wrong person.
- Administering the wrong day.
- All medication not coming out of the blister pack because it is stuck to the inside of the pack or has caught up in the foil.
- Administering at wrong times.
- Not seeing the service user take and swallow the medication.
- Not acting on messages in handover or communication regarding medication review.
- Knowing that you haven't given out the medication and not doing anything to correct this.

13.6.8 Reasons for errors when administering medication

The following are some of the reasons errors occur if you fail to follow the guidelines:

- Got distracted.
- Did not know routine.
- Check not done, or done incorrectly.

- Thinking that someone had done it.
- Not passing information on to other members of staff at handover time.
- Forgot.
- Did not check what must be given.
- Did not check, pushed the wrong day.
- Did not check the name or person being given medication.
- Lack of knowledge: you *must* take action if you know an error has occurred.
- Did not check medication before blister pack was broken and after medication has been given to the service user.
- Can't tell time, did not read the MAR sheet.
- Not following the procedure, being distracted.
- Forgot, overlooked, or did not act immediately.

All the above errors are preventable and so should not occur. However, if they do occur you must immediately inform the shift leader, manager on duty or the out-of-hours on-call manager or call the paramedics by dialling 999.

13.7   Medication best practice checklist

- Read the guidelines and always follow them.
- Always keep medicines in the same place in the cabinet.
- Keep bottles clean – wipe them if sticky or dirty.
- Lock the medication cabinet when not in use.
- When you run out of tablets or any medication, replace with a new supply from the medication store.
- Do not allow yourself to be distracted while you are in the medication administration process.
- Never leave medication intended for one person, unattended in the presence of other service users.

13.8   Learning outcomes

On completion of this chapter coupled with the practical induction by a senior member of staff in the organisation you working for, you should possess the knowledge, skills and experience required to administer, store and document medication handled on behalf of the service users

13.9   Framework for reflective practice

➤ *Knowledge:*   What have you learnt from reading this chapter?
➤ *Skills:*   What do you know, or can do differently now, that you did not/could not do before reading this chapter?
➤ *Practices:*   How can you perform a task now better than before?

13.10 References

British Medical Association (2011) *New Guide to Medication and Drugs*, 8th edn. London: Dorling Kindersley.

British National Formulary (BNF). http://www.bnf.org.uk/bnf/

Cooper, B. and Gerlis, L. (2003) *A Consumer's Guide to Prescription Medicines*. London: Bounty Books.

Department of Health (1999) *Clinical Governance: Quality in the New NHS*. HSC 1999/065. London: DoH.

Dougherty, L. and Lister, S. (2008) *The Royal Marsden Hospital Manual of Clinical Nursing Procedures*, 7th edn. Oxford: Wiley-Blackwell.

National Prescribing Centre (2009) A Guide to Good Practice in the Management of Controlled Drugs in Primary Care (England), 3rd edn. www.npc.co.uk

Nursing & Midwifery Council (2004) *Guidelines for the Administration of Medicines 2004*. www.nmc-uk.org.

Nursing & Midwifery Council (2009) *Guidelines for Records and Record Keeping*. www.nmc-uk.org.

Nursing & Midwifery Council (2010) *Standards for Medicines Management*. www.nmc-uk.org.

Parragon Book Services Ltd (1996) *Medicines: The Comprehensive Guide*. Parragon Book Services Ltd.

Royal Pharmaceutical Society of Great Britain (2007) *The Handling of Medicines in Social Care*. www.rpsgb.org.uk

Skills for Care (2010) *Knowledge Set for Medication*. www.skillsforcare.org.uk

Legislation

Data Protection Act 1998

Disability Discrimination Act 1995 as amended

Human Rights Act 1998

The Medicines Act 1968

The Mental Capacity Act 2005

The Misuse of Drugs Act 1971

The Misuse of Drugs (Safe Custody) Regulations 1973

National Health Service and Community Care Act 1990

The Shipman Inquiry 2005

13.11 Induction workbook

1. What is a blister pack?

   _____

   _____

2. How is medication recorded and where is the information stored?

   _____

   _____

3. What would you do if you found any medication on the floor?

   _____

   _____

4. Why is it important that medication procedures are routinely followed?

   _____

   _____

5. Who is responsible for ordering medication and recording the delivery?

    _____

    _____

6. What are the two main statutes of law in medicines?

    _____

    _____

7. Why is it important to wear gloves when handling medication in tablet form?

    _____

    _____

8. What would be the procedure for disposing 'out of date/use' medication?

    _____

    _____

9. What is the importance of an MAR sheet in relation to the service provider?

    _____

    _____

10. Outline ten tips for safe administration of medication in any home/project.

    _____

    _____

11. What procedure should you follow once you realise a medication error has occurred?

    _____

    _____

12. List the possible medication errors that are likely to occur in a home where there are more than two service users.

    _____

    _____

13. List the possible errors that occur when administering medication and their causes.

    _____

    _____

14. Outline the legislations associated with the control and management of medication in care settings.

    _____

    _____

14   Moving and Handling

AIMS
- To optimise person and handler safety without compromising the person's mobility and care needs
- To be able to describe the responsibilities of employees and employers
- To identify the types of hazards in relation to moving and handling
- To describe how risks can be controlled and eliminated
- To be able to recognise legal aspects in moving and handling
- To show how to work toward the safest, ergonomically suitable environment for moving and handling

14.1   Introduction

Definitions that apply to moving and handling:
- Any transporting or supporting of a load (including the lifting, putting down, pushing, pulling, carrying or moving thereof) by hand or by bodily force.
- Manual handling includes both transporting a load and supporting a load in a static posture. The load may be moved or supported by the hands or any other part of the body — for example, the shoulder.
- Manual handling also includes the intentional dropping of a load and the throwing of a load, whether into a receptacle or from one person to another. (The Manual Handling Operations Regulations)

14.2   Types of moving and handling

14.2.1   Service user handling

- The moving of or assisting to move a service user from one place to another.
- The supporting of a service user, as in the whole body or in part (i.e. a limb) and the transporting of a service user in a chair, bed, trolley or hoist.

14.2.2   Static loads

- The moving or supporting of any inanimate load, e.g. a box of office stationary.

14.2.3   Therapeutic manual handling

- The specialist manual handling manoeuvres and transfers that needs to be performed by therapists, nurses and other staff to assist in the service user's rehabilitation.

14.3   Risk assessment in manual handling

- An assessment of risk is a careful examination of what, in the workplace, could cause harm to people, so that employers can decide whether they have taken enough precautions or whether more should be done to prevent harm.

- The aim is to make sure that no one gets hurt by anticipating foreseeable risks.
- Where a hazardous moving and handling operation cannot be avoided, a thorough assessment must be undertaken, and measures must be introduced to reduce the risk of injury to the lowest level reasonably practicable
- Community staff and others who work in the service users' own home *are* covered by Health and Safety laws.
- Home workers should not be expected to manually lift service users on their own, without a moving and handling assessment being completed.
- Where necessary special arrangements should be made.

14.4   Basic legislation that govern all manual handling tasks

Manual handling is covered by the following legislation:

- The Health and Safety at Work Act 1974 covers the general health and safety duties of employers and employees.
- The Manual Handling Operations Regulations 1992 requires employers to avoid hazardous manual handling and, where this is not possible, to assess and eliminate or reduce the risks of manual handling. They also require employees to cooperate fully with the steps their employers take to meet these regulations
- The European Community regulations, which came into force in December 1992, require all staff to be trained in lifting techniques and risk assessment and *not* to attempt to lift anything or manoeuvre anyone without the necessary basic instructions and practice.

Employers' responsibilities of moving and handling are to:

- successfully implement and monitor compliance with the policy in the areas for which they are responsible;
- ensure moving and handling risk assessments are carried out within each work area as appropriate, and for each service user upon admission to an in-patient unit/home/housing project;
- ensure that moving and handling assessment are a basis for action to minimise moving and handling and thereby reduce the risk of injury to staff, service users and carers;
- ensure that staff are aware that they do not participate in moving of service users or inanimate objects until they have received training in safe handling and training in the use of equipment;
- ensure that risk assessment for the handling of inanimate loads are reviewed at regular intervals or if the situation changes;
- ensure that moving and handling equipment is available and used where risk assessment identifies risk to staff and or the service user;
- ensure that all staff enrols on the mandatory training programme where appropriate moving and handling will be facilitated by the external/internal trainers/workshops;
- ensure that staff are trained locally in the use of moving and handling equipment;
- check that the methods of moving and handling used are appropriate to their environment and occupation and in line with training received;

- ensure that staff are aware of their responsibility to check that moving and handling equipment is in good order immediately prior to use (e.g. slings have been checked and are in good repair);
- ensure that all moving and handing incidents are reported using the incident report form and appropriate investigations are carried out;
- ensure that details of moving and handling equipment are recorded on the home/project device inventory;
- be assured that mechanical moving and handling equipment and lifting accessories are checked/serviced by a registered competent contractor at six-monthly intervals (Lifting Operations and Lifting Equipment Regulations (LOLER) and Provision and Use of Work Equipment Regulations (PUWER));
- ensure that local arrangements exist for the checking of slings and harnesses by staff prior to use; check that the safe working load (SWL) is clearly visible on service user hoists;
- ensure that wheels on trolleys are in good working order;
- take into account and where necessary re-access an individual's ability to use control methods developed from a moving and handling assessment where the individual is a new expectant mother and keep the assessment under regular review;
- re-assess individual capabilities where a member of staff is returning from sick leave as a result of a work-based moving and handling injury or following pregnancy prior to the individual carrying out moving and handling activity.

14.5   Specific requirements for service users in care setting

- On admission all service users should have a personal profile of their mobility status and a moving and handling assessment should be completed.
- Using the organisation's documentation policy, information should be kept in a prominent position within the health care records and reviewed at regular intervals or where service user requirements have changed.
- The employer should ensure that staff are aware of the service user moving and handling risk assessment and care plan.
- Service users should be encouraged and where appropriate receive training in personal moving and handling techniques.
- Staff should be instructed in the use of service user hoists, and records of such training should be retained.

14.5.1   Responsibilities of the employer

1. The employer's duty is to avoid manual handling as far as reasonably practicable if there is a possibility of injury.
2. If this cannot be done then they must reduce the risk of injury as far as reasonably practicable.
3. If an employee is complaining of discomfort, any changes to work to avoid or reduce manual handling must be monitored to check they are having a positive effect. However, if they are not working satisfactorily, alternatives must be considered.

Manual handling regulations require an employer, in consultation with employees, to:

- ensure that plant, work practices and the work environment are designed to eliminate manual handling injuries;
- identify the manual handling tasks that may place a worker at risks;
- assess the level of risk to workers carrying out that task;
- introduce measures to control those risks;
- review what has been done.

14.5.2 Employees' responsibilities in moving and handling

- It is the responsibility of employees to take reasonable care of their own health and safety and that of others who may be affected by their actions or lack of it.
- They must communicate with their employers so that they too are able to meet their health and safety duties.
- They must carry out risk assessments in accordance with instruction and training.
- They must not expose themselves or others to significant risk from moving and handling operations.
- They must not participate in moving and handling of service users until training has been provided nor use equipment (e.g. hoists) without the relevant training.
- They must work within the risk assessment using the correct moving and handling methods indicated by training and by individual capability.
- They must attend training on an annual basis in moving and handling as part of the mandatory training.
- They must ensure that they are fit to undertake moving and handling tasks. Any change in health that may affect ability to undertake moving and handling operations should be reported to the line manager.
- They must check that equipment is in good working order before use, ensuring that it has an up-to-date service validation date attached to the equipment.
- They must use equipment provided in accordance with training provided and in accordance to manufacturer's instructions.
- They must not use equipment for lifting or moving a service user that does not have a safe working load (SWL) clearly marked and must ensure that the lifting is within the capacity of the equipment.
- They must ensure that clothing and footwear is suitable for safe moving and handling practice. For example robust flat footwear and clothing which allows the adoption of good posture.
- They must report any problems or concerns in respect of equipment for moving and handling to the project/home manager.
- They must be aware of plans to deal with service users whose weight exceeds that of the weight capacity of standard issue equipment, i.e. hoists, slings and beds.
- They must report circumstances when safe-lifting methods cannot be used or where circumstances have changed, increasing the risk of injury.
- They must encourage service users' independence and mobilisation, where appropriate.

14.5.3 Agency and bank staff

Agency and bank staff should be regarded as employees for the purpose of compliance with arrangements for moving and handling. Employees have general health and safety duties to:

- adhere to and follow appropriate systems of work laid down for their safety;
- apply any manual handling training they have been given and comply with reasonable instructions on the performance of manual handling tasks;
- make proper use of equipment provided for their safety;
- cooperate with their employer on health and safety matters;
- inform the employer if they identify hazardous handling activities;
- take care to ensure that their activities do not put them or others at risk.

14.6 Meaning and purpose of risk assessment in relation to moving and handling

Know what could put you at risk. When assessing the move, staff should consider the following aspects of any handling job.

14.6.1 The task

- Will it involve twisting or stretching?
- Poor posture such as stooping?
- Risk sudden movement?
- Frequent or prolonged physical effort?
- Insufficient rest or recovery time? (All the above increase the risk of injury.)

14.6.2 Your capabilities

- Will the move require unusual strength?
- Will it pose a risk to your health condition (including pregnancy)?
- Will it require special knowledge or training?

14.6.3 The working environment

- Are space problems hindering safe movement?
- Are floors slippery or uneven?
- Are there different floor levels?
- Is lighting too poor to see what you need to see?

14.6.4 The load or person

Ask yourself if the load or the person will be unstable, too heavy, too bulky or too difficult to grasp.

14.7   Basic rules for safe handling

The following are the basic rules to develop a skill that will enable you to handle loads easily, effectively and safely.

14.7.1   Planning

- First size up the job.
- Choose a clear route
- Decide how you intend to do it.
- Check access and that destination is clear and free from hazards.
- Assess where to hold the load relative to the centre of gravity.
- Check for sharps.

14.7.2   Advice and precautions

1. Check the weight – do not attempt *too much* by yourself, get help.
2. Alternatives – use handling aids where provided and it is safe to do so.
3. Protection: Wear and use protective clothing and safety equipment appropriate to the work.
4. Correct posture:
   - As you lift, tuck in your chin, this will help for a straight back.
   - Keep the load and your arms close to the body to avoid strain.
5. Use the legs to power the lift – if the load is to be moved to another level, then bend your knees, not your back. Keep your back straight.
6. Body weight – use your body as a counterweight to reduce muscular effort.
7. Feet position – place your feet slightly apart, one slightly ahead, pointing in the direction you intend to go.
8. Use your eyes – look where you are going.
9. Correct grip – get a good *firm* grip, not just your fingertips.
10. Set a good example – let the service users and others see you get it right.

14.7.3   General information on manual handling

If you find someone on the floor:

- *do not* attempt to lift him or her on your own;
- in the first instance check to see that they are 'safe';
- if they are unconscious, they should be turned into recovery position;
- summon assistance;
- if they are bleeding, it is stopped;
- no service user should be assisted off the floor;
- if the service user is conscious, ask if they are in pain;
- if the service user cannot get themselves up, you must call an ambulance, you should *never* lift them as they may have fractures.

14.8 Use of correct moving and handling equipment

14.8.1 Make use of simple aids

When moving and handling a person or load be sure to have proper training before using any handling aid. Ensure the equipment is in good working order.

14.8.2 Types of simple aids

1. *Small transfer boards and sliding boards*

These can be used to transfer a person from one level surface to another (for example, from bed to wheelchair).

2. *Sliding sheets*

- These can be used to move a person who is lying down from one surface to another of the same height, from hospital trolley to a bed in conjunction with a transfer board.
- They can also be used to move a person up and down the bed.
- They can be used to reposition a supine service user.
- They can be used to turn a sitting person towards the side of the bed, or in conjunction with a transfer board.

3. *Turning disc and turntables*

- On the floor, these may be used with care to rotate or pivot a standing person.
- On a seat or a bed, they can be used to rotate a person to face the side of a bed or the inside of a car

4. *Using hoists*

There are three main types of hoists:

- Tracked overhead hoist: these provide independence, since the person being moved can operate the equipment alone, once they have been set up. They are safe way to move a person over a longer distance.
- Fixed hoists: these are useful when overhead tracks cannot be installed, and are ideal for short distances.
- Mobile hoists: these are very versatile and can help move a person in and out of a vehicle or to different locations in the home, for example from the bedroom to the lounge.

14.8.3 Types of slings

It is important to note that using the correct sling is essential for hoist safety. There are three major types of slings:

1. *Hammock*

- These provide all-round support and comfort.

- They can be used without the person actively assisting in the move.

2. *Divided leg*

- These are simple to use and may be applied with the person in a sitting position.

3. *Independent*

- These require a person to have good upper-body control.
- They are easy for removal of clothes to aid toileting and cleaning.

14.8.4 Basic guidelines to use hoists safely

- Only use equipment that you are properly trained and competent to use.
- Always follow the manufacturer's instructions and review them before using any mechanical aid.
- Choose the right hoist and sling, based on the assessment. Be sure it is the best one for you and the person being moved and the task involved.
- Make sure the hoists and the slings are compatible – use the correct sling for the hoist and the correct size for the service user.
- Check the maximum weight limits of the equipment with the person's weight.
- Check for hazards such as wet floors or blocked paths.
- Always be prepared for the unexpected, such as sudden movement triggered by a Tonic Clonic seizure.
- Don't take chances – move slowly and steadily.
- Avoid manual lifting whenever possible.
- Remember you have other options.

14.9   For safety and comfort before, during and after the move

To ensure the person's safety and comfort it is important to consult their care plan. Then follow these guidelines.

14.9.1   Before the move

- Explain what you are going to do and what the person can expect.
- Ask the person about any special needs or wishes.
- Make the necessary adjustments to the equipment.
- Tuck in any loose clothes.

14.9.2   During the move

- Encourage the person to help with the move, if appropriate.
- Constantly monitor the equipment and check the person for comfort and safety.
- Keep a sharp lookout for hazards.
- Reassure the person as you go along.

14.9.3 After the move

- Secure the equipment.
- Check any wounds, drips, splints etc. and check that clothes are comfortable.
- Ask if the person needs any other help (e.g. putting on shoes).
- Thank him or her for cooperating with the move.

14.9.4 Apply the principles of moving

When (moving) working with people, first check the person's care plan and manual handling risk assessment.

1. *Evaluate the situation*

- Make sure you are aware of what you have to do.
- Confirm that you have the necessary equipment and people to help.
- Ensure the person is well enough to be moved.

2. *Tell the person*

- Explain what you are going to do.
- The person will be more relaxed and able to cooperate.
- Encourage the person to help with the move, if appropriate.

3. *Position the equipment*

- Provide any equipment (for example, trapeze) that may help the person assist in the move.
- Prepare moving aids and hoist.
- Position wheelchairs and stretchers as close to the person as possible.

4. *Make necessary adjustments*

- Adjust the chair or stretcher to bed level or vice versa and lower any hand rails. This will reduce the amount of moving required.
- Be sure to lock the wheels on the chair and the bed.

5. *Don't take chances*

- Use only those procedures with which you are familiar.
- Guessing the correct procedures, improvising, or failing to exercise proper caution may mean danger to you or the person you are moving.
- Keep your knowledge up to date by attending refresher courses and sourcing out new information on moving and handling.

6. *Get help if you need help*

- Don't hesitate to ask questions or seek help if you are not sure of the procedure or your ability to handle the situation.
- It is better to be safe than to be sorry.

14.10 Moving and handling of service users

- Always consider whether it is necessary to move and handle a service user.
- In some instances it may be appropriate to encourage the service user to move themselves under close supervision.
- Do not carry out any moving and handling that would put the service user, you or your colleague at risk of harm.
- Prepare the handling area and ensure that it is safe and free from obstruction.
- Always assess before commencing a moving and handling task.
- Always select the appropriate moving and handling action/equipment for the task.
- Keep the service user/load to be moved as close to your body as possible.
- Explain the moving and handling action to the service user about to be moved and also to a colleague who may be assisting.
- Test your grip and the weight if necessary before attempting the moving and handling action. Be self-aware, know your own capabilities and do not exceed them.
- Identify a leader prior to moving and handling.
- The moving and handling lead must give clear precise instructions (e.g. ready, steady lift).
- Always lift within the accepted weight limits.
- Do not carry out a moving and handling task if it is unsafe to do so.
- If equipment is required always check that it is in good working order and the safe working load (SWL) is adhered to.
- Always consider the ergonomic principles.

Caution: Never manual lift unless you have no other option – always ask 'Do I need to lift?'

NB: if the person cannot or will not cooperate with the move, speak to your manager or a team leader and re-assess the situation.

14.10.1 Moving and handling during emergency situations

- In emergency situations, e.g. fire, it may be necessary to manually handle people to a place of safety as a matter of urgency. Employees should always use the best practical means of moving and handling without compromising the saving of life.
- Where a service user is observed to fall whilst staff are present, staff should first look after their own health, safety and welfare. They should refrain from the natural tendency to catch the service user to stop them from falling.
- In such circumstances they should:

  o allow the service user to fall naturally unless they are in danger, in which case, it would be appropriate to nudge them out of harm's way;
  o ensure that the service user's head is protected from trauma, so far as is reasonably practicable.

- Where a service user is discovered on the floor already, staff should refrain from any attempt to immediately move the service user. In such circumstances, they should:

  o examine the service user for injury and make them comfortable;
  o assess the most appropriate means of moving the service user back to their bed or chair, this may include:
  o advising the service user how to get up;
  o using, with colleagues assistance, an appropriate sling and hoist.

- If control and restraint are to be undertaken in an emergency situation, staff must adhere to the techniques demonstrated in the control and restraint training programme.
- Foreseeable emergencies must be assessed and have planned safe systems of work in place.

14.11 Learning outcomes

- To gain awareness of employer and employee responsibilities under relevant National Health & Safety legislation including most recent versions of the Manual Handling Regulations and the Display Screen Equipment (DSE) Regulations.
- To gain awareness of responsibilities under local Policies for Manual Handling, Display Screen Equipment and Management of Health and Safety at Work 1974.
- To gain awareness of where additional advice and information can be sought relating to manual handling issues if necessary.
- To acquire the ability to conduct 'on the spot' risk assessments prior to moving and handling service users and non-patient loads.
- To acquire the ability to conduct 'on the spot' Display Screen Equipment (DSE) workstation risk assessments where appropriate.
- To gather the knowledge of:
  o an ergonomic approach to manual handling and other work tasks leading to improved working posture;
  o good back care including general musculoskeletal health.
- To gain awareness of risk management processes and safe systems of work within the organisation.
- To acquire the ability to provide service users with the best quality care using appropriate, safe and dignified moving and handling procedures

14.12 Framework for reflective practice

➢ *Knowledge:* What have you learnt from reading this chapter?
➢ *Skills:* What do you know, or can do differently now, that you did not/could not do before reading this chapter?
➢ *Practices:* How can you perform a task now better than before?

14.13 References

Control of Substances Hazard to Health Regulations (COSHH) 2002.

Disability Discrimination Act (DDA) 1998.
Health and Safety at Work etc. Act 1974.
Human Rights Act 2001.
Lifting Operations and Lifting Equipment Regulations 1998.
Management of Health and Safety at Work 1992 (amended 1999).
Manual Handling Regulations 1992 (amended 2002) & guidelines L23 (available at www.hse.gov.uk/foi/internalops/fod/oc/300-399/313_5.pdf).
NHS and Community Care Act 1980.
Personal Protection Equipment at Work Regulations (PPE) 1992.
Provision and Use of Work Equipment Regulations, 1998.
Reporting of Injuries, Diseases and Dangerous Occurrences Regulations (RIDDOR) 1995.
Smith, J. and Lloyd, P. (2004) *Guide to the Handling of People*, 5th edn. Back Care in collaboration with the Royal College of Nursing and the National Back Exchange (http://www.nationalbackexchange.org).
Work Equipment Regulations 1998.
Workplace (Health Safety and Welfare) Regulations 1992.

14.14 Induction workbook

1. List the five areas of the spine and their functions.

    _____

    _____

2. Outline the current legislation that governs moving and handling.

    _____

    _____

3. Explain what risk assessment is in relation to moving and handling.

    _____

    _____

4. Outline the principles of correct moving and handling.

    _____

    _____

5. What are your responsibilities and the role of others in relation to maintaining a safe environment?

    _____

    _____

6. Describe situations that may be a risk to you when it comes to moving and handling and how you can avoid them.

    _____

    _____

15 Fire Safety

AIMS
- To explain how fires start and how to prevent them starting
- To advise on how to raise the alarm in the event of a fire
- To show how to identify different types of extinguishers
- To explain how to extinguish fires
- To advise on what other actions to take in the event of a fire

15.1 Introduction

Fire is clearly destructive and dangerous to both people and properties and the environment.

- In the outbreak of a fire it is essential that the correct procedures are in place and followed to ensure safety of those affected.
- No matter what kind of work you do, you need to make every effort to keep the service users and yourself safe.
- Safety is everyone's responsibility.

15.2 Fire prevention measures

Measures to be taken to prevent fire from starting in a project/home/residential setting or care environment:

15.2.1 Risk assessment

Assessments should include:

- identifying hazards and people at risk including those with disabilities;
- removing or reducing the hazards and managing the remaining risks to acceptable levels;
- contacting your local fire service to visit and give safety advice and talk to both the staff and service users.

15.2.2 Project / care setting safety

- The manager or team leader should act as the fire warden for the project/residential setting and be responsible for the evacuation of the premises in the event of fire and fire drills.
- The manager should ensure that regular fire alarms tests take place (weekly), escape lighting checks (monthly) and evacuation drills (quarterly) are carried out and records kept.

15.2.3 Training/awareness

- The project/residential managers must ensure that all staff are, and remain, familiar with the relevant fire and emergency procedures for the project/residential/supported living schemes/care setting.
- Managers should also arrange for staff training that may be appropriate (e.g. using fire blanket, what type of fire extinguishers to be used on what types of fire, i.e. electricity, gas, wood etc.).

15.3 General fire safety guidelines

15.3.1 Upon discovering a fire

- Raise the alarm immediately by shouting 'fire' or breaking the fire glass panels located in the house.
- Do not tackle the fire if this would put you at risk.
- Use appliances provided (extinguishers, fire blankets etc.).
- If you do tackle the fire (where applicable *only* if appropriately trained or safe to do so).

15.3.2 On hearing a fire alarm (or being notified of fire)

- Call the fire bridge immediately.
- Leave the building by the nearest safe exit and report at the relevant assembly point.
- Do not run – exit the building swiftly.
- Do not stop to collect personal belongings.
- Do not re-enter the building unless authorised to do so.
- Do inform the person in charge if you suspect someone is still in the building.

15.3.3 Electrics

- Always use an electrical circuit breaker (residual current device – RCD) with any appliance – such as vacuum cleaner, electrical kettle etc.
- Check for signs of loose wiring and faulty plugs and sockets.
- Replace any worn or taped-up cables and leads.
- Don't overload sockets.
- Don't put cables under carpets or mats.
- Check the maximum amps that the fuse in a plug can handle.
- Turn off equipment and unplug it when not in use. Store it in a safe place.
- If you need to use an adapter, ensure it has a fuse and keep the total output to no more than 13 amps.

15.3.4 Kitchens

- Keep electrical leads and items that can catch fire easily away from cookers, toasters etc. dish clothes, kitchen towels etc.
- Keep electrical leads and appliances away from water.

- Keep ovens, toasters, hobs and grills clean – a build-up of crumbs, fat and grease can easily catch fire.
- Ensure saucepan handles don't stick out when on the hot hobs, always face them inward.
- Keep a fire blanket in the kitchen.
- Don't overfill chips pans (more than half full of oil).

15.3.5 Chips pan fires

- Only tackle fire if you are sure you can put out the fire and stay safe.
- Turn off the heat if safe to do so.
- Do not move the pan.
- Cover the flaming pan with a damp (not wet) cloth. Put a fire blanket over the pan if you have one
- Never throw water over the hot pan – the oil will explode

15.3.6 Cigarettes

- Always use proper ashtrays.
- Empty ashtrays often.
- Ensure cigarettes are properly extinguished.
- Never smoke in bed.
- Take extra care if smoking whilst drowsy, taking prescription medication or drinking.
- Keep matches/lighters out of the reach of children.
- Follow the care plan guidelines for lighters and smoking

15.3.7 Candles

- Never leave candles unattended.
- Put them out completely at night.
- Place them on heat resistant surfaces.
- Keep them away from anything that may catch fire (curtains etc.).
- Keep out of reach of children and pets.

15.3.8 Be prepared

Everybody affected should be aware of what to do and how to escape in the event of fire.

- Escape routes should be planned and exits kept clear. Keep doors and window keys handy, where applicable.
- Ensure fire safety risk assessment is conducted and reviewed at least annually or when need arises.
- Ensure that regular fire alarms tests are carried out weekly, emergency lighting checks monthly and evacuation drills are carried out quarterly.
- Make sure all relevant fire exit and evacuation signs are in place.
- Test smoke alarm batteries regularly (where applicable).

- Consider how anyone with restricted mobility (e.g. a wheelchair user) or other disability would evacuate the building.
- If a fire starts and there is smoke, keep low where the air is clearer.
- Keep fire doors closed to prevent fire from spreading.

15.3.9 Help service users prepare for an emergency

- Teach the service users what to do in case of a fire.
- Practise a fire escape plan together.
- Keep escape paths clear. Remove clutter or furniture that could blocks exit doors and pathways.

15.3.10 Know how to respond in the event of a fire

- Stay calm – and help service users to stay calm.
- Help service users leave the building using the nearest exit.
- Alert everyone in the house by shouting fire or breaking the fire glass panels to sound the alarm.
- Contact the fire brigade from a neighbour's house or a mobile phone.
- Keep a head count for all service users and staff.
- If you are unable to remove a service user, keep the fire door shut and get help as soon as possible – do not put yourself at risk.

15.3.11 If the escape route is blocked

- You may be able to escape from a window if you are on ground or first floor – only consider this option as a last resort.
- Don't jump. Lower yourself from the ledge before dropping – this should break your fall.
- Where possible throw beddings, cushions etc. outside to break your fall.
- Shut the doors and use beddings and clothes to block the bottom of the door, this should prevent smoke from entering the room if it's not a fire door.
- If you can't escape from the building through windows get everyone into one room (probably with a telephone and a window).
- Shout for help from the window if necessary.
- Avoid opening the fire doors as they are meant to keep smoke out and air (wind) which help accelerate the fire.
- Lean out of the window to breathe if you have to from time to time.

15.3.12 If your clothes catch fire

- Don't run around – this will only fuel the flames.
- Lie down and roll – it smothers the flames, which makes it harder for the fire to spread and helps protect your face and (head) hair (flames burn upwards).
- Smother the flames by covering them with heavy material like a coat or blanket.
- Remember the basic principles when on fire – *stop! drop! and roll!*

15.4   Learning outcomes

- To be able to recount the main causes of fire and to recount the potential for active staff involvement in fire prevention in the workplace.
- To be able to recount the steps required when discovering a fire in the buildings, including how to initiate the emergency response.
- To be able to recount the necessary steps to be taken when hearing the fire alarm sound.
- To be able to state, in broad terms, how to evacuate service users at risk to a place of relative safety, where applicable.
- To be able to inform other staff, service users and visitors to the social and healthcare environment of any basic fire safety issues and to be able to direct them to the local fire marshal or warden if any further clarification is necessary.
- To be able to demonstrate your knowledge of the difference between relevant equipment and its usage, if appropriate. For example, by matching particular fire types and the most appropriate fire extinguisher.
- To be able to identify areas of arson risk and the associated importance of good housekeeping.

15.5   Framework for reflective practice

- ➤ *Knowledge:*   What have you learnt from reading this chapter?
- ➤ *Skills:*   What do you know, or can do differently now, that you did not/could not do before reading this chapter?
- ➤ *Practices:*   How can you perform a task now better than before?

15.6   References

Building Regulations 2000.
Electrical Safety Council: Top tips on electrical safety: http://www.esc.org.uk
Fire and Rescue Services Act 2004.
Fire Precautions (Factories, Offices, Shops and Railway Premises) Order 1989.
Fire Precautions Act 1971 (Modifications) (Revocation) Regulations 1989.
Health and Safety (Training for Employment) Regulations 1990.
Health and Safety at Work Act etc. 1974.
HM Government – Fire Safety Risk Assessment: 'Means of Escape for Disabled People'.
HM Government – Fire Safety Risk Assessment: 'Healthcare Premises'.
Housing Act 2004.
Management of Health and Safety at Work and Fire Precautions (Workplace) (Amendment) Regulations 2003.
Management of Health and Safety at Work Regulations 1999.
NHS Executive: HTM Firecode suite of guidance documents.
Regulatory Reform (Fire Safety) Order 2005.
Reporting of Injuries, Diseases and Dangerous Occurrences Regulations (RIDDOR) 1995.
Safety Representatives and Safety Committees Regulations 1977.

15.7 Induction workbook

1. Outline practices to prevent fires from starting.

    _____
    _____

2. Explain four ways in which you can prevent a fire from spreading:

    i.   _____

    ii.   _____
          _____
          _____
    iii. _____
          _____

3. Describe methods of allowing service users and staff to understand and follow emergency procedures in the event of a fire.

    _____
    _____

4. Outline the procedures to prevent fire.

    _____
    _____

5. Outline and demonstrate emergency procedure in the event of a fire.

    _____
    _____

16 Infection Control

AIMS

- To have the insight to improve best standards of infection control
- To identify areas of good and poor practice in infection control
- To understand the chain of infection and how to break it
- To have an increased awareness of infection control considerations within non-acute healthcare settings

16.1 Introduction

One of the essential knowledge requirements of a health and social care worker is that of how to prevent and control infection.

- It is important that health and social care workers consistently practise infection control techniques to ensure the health and safety of service users, themselves and others (health professionals, families or friends) who may be present in the residential or care environment.

16.2 Legislation and legal requirements

- The Care Standards Act 2000 and Associated Regulations (2002)
- Health and Safety at Work Act (1974)

    The Act states that the employer has a duty of care towards employees, service users and others who visit hospital/care home/care environment. Employers are expected to develop their own infection control policy which outlines the procedures as follows:

    o 'It shall be the duty of every employer to ensure, so far as reasonably practicable, the health, safety and welfare at work of all his/her employees.' The employer is required to provide appropriate information and instruction with the appropriate safety equipment, training and supervision to ensure that their employees are protected at work.
    o Employees must comply with any safety policies or procedures put in place to protect their health.
    o Employees must also protect their own health and safety by using any protective clothing issued to them.
    o Employees also have a duty to make sure that their actions do not harm the health and safety of others.

- Environmental Protection Act (1990)
- Environmental Protection (Duty of Care) Regulations (1991)
- Control of Substances Hazardous to Health Regulations – COSHH (1999)

These regulations apply to all workplace hazardous substances (including micro-organisms) and encourage the limitation of exposure to hazardous substances. They also recommend the use of personal protective equipment such as gloves, gowns and aprons where necessary.

- Occupiers Liability Act (1957)
- Reporting of Injuries, Diseases and Dangerous Occurrences Regulations – RIDDOR (1995)
- Public Health Control of Disease Act (1984)
- Public Health Infectious Disease Regulations (1988)
- Food Safety Act (1990)

16.3   What is an infection?

An infection is the invasion of the body tissues by disease-causing organisms, e.g. bacteria or viruses; such micro-organisms are found in, around and on people and their surroundings at all times. (en.wikipedia.org/wiki/Infection)

Micro-organisms that cause infections are known as pathogens. They are classified as:

- Bacteria – these are classified into different groups and can be pathogenic. They are susceptible to a greater or lesser extent to antibiotics, e.g. S*taphylococcal aureus* (found nearly everywhere in the environment, i.e. soil, air).
- Virus – a virus is much smaller than bacteria and can survive out of the body for a time. Viruses are not susceptible to antibiotics although anti-viral drugs are available, e.g. Acyclovir. Most viral infections are self-limiting.
- Pathogenic fungi – can either be moulds or yeast. An example of mould that can cause infection in humans is *Trichophytyon rubrum* – which is one cause of ringworm. Another example is *Candida albicans*, commonly called Thrush.
- Protozoa – microscopic free living organisms, e.g. *Giardia lamblia* which causes diarrhoea.
- Parasites – some are pathogenic and cause infection and are spread from person to person, e.g. scabies.
- Prions – are infectious protein particles, e.g. the prion causing (New) Variant Creutzfeldt-Jakob disease.

16.4   The spread of infection

- Given the right conditions – warmth, dampness and darkness – bacteria and viruses multiply rapidly and can cause diseases which at first may affect some and often all parts of the body, e.g. cholera, cold/flu, salmonella via chicken, or malaria via insects bites – mosquito.
- The immune system comprises white cells, which fight infection, but often in doing so cause symptoms such as redness, swelling, heat and pain and loss of function (locally) and feverishness (generally).

- The immune system can be weakened with age and even destroyed completely and therefore be unable to resist a virulent infection. Infection by micro-organism will more easily take place in someone whose resistance is weakened, e.g. by age, nutrition or the effects of drugs.
- Certain groups of service users/patients are at increased risk of acquiring an infection because their body's defence mechanism may be weakened by certain types of medication.
- In most elderly people there are chests or urinary infections, both of which will cause the individuals to be unwell, possibly feverish and confused.
- Urinary infections will cause the urine to be dark in colour and have an unpleasant odour.
- Another common infection amongst elderly people is cellulitis, which occur when ulcers and wounds become infected. In all cases, medical advice should be sought promptly.
- Infection is not only a problem for the elderly: all groups of service users can suffer from infection.

16.5   Factors responsible for infection

Many of the factors responsible for the increase in infection rates are well understood in the care environment, enabling the development of strategies to support infection prevention and control.

The basis of these strategies lies in understanding how infection is transmitted. This is now commonly known as the chain of infection.

16.5.1   The chain of infection

The chain of infection describes the sequence of events involved in the spread of infection as a series of interconnecting links. Prevention and control of infection can be aimed towards breaking these links, thereby interrupting the chain and preventing the spread of infection.

- An infectious agent can be any micro-organism capable of producing disease, including viruses and bacteria. They can be from the service user/patient/staff or acquired from an external source.
- The reservoir describes the environment in which a micro-organism can survive. Places, people and equipment can all act as reservoirs.
- The portal exit is the route by which the micro-organism leaves the reservoir. This can be by excretion or secretion of body fluids, in droplets, or on skin. (In addition the placenta acts as a portal exit in the transmission of infection from mother to foetus).
- The means of transmission describes the way in which a micro-organism is acquired and can be considered as contact transmission (via direct or in-direct contact), droplets transmission or airborne transmission.
- Of the six links in the chain of infection, the means of transmission is the easiest to break and is, therefore the key to cross-infection control within the health and social care environment.
- The portal of entry is the route by which the infectious agents gains access to the susceptible host, and is often the same as the port of exit.
- The susceptible host is the final link in the chain of infection.

Ninety per cent of germs on the hands are found under the nails, and the number of bacteria can double in 20 minutes. After one day without washing hands a single bacterium can multiply by two billion. These bugs can cause diarrhoea, fever and other nasty illness (Woodburn and Mackenzie, 2004).

16.6   Signs of infection

- looking flushed and feeling feverish;
- localised swelling, redness or discharge;
- enlarged glands of the neck, armpits or groin;
- pain;
- listlessness and lack of appetite;
- a change in behaviour perhaps agitation, restlessness aggressive or confusion.

The care worker should ensure that the service user with an infection has:

- had medical attention;
- good fluid intake to prevent dehydration;
- clothing changes or room temperature adjustment to a lower or higher temperature;
- comfort;
- rest.

16.7   Hand washing

When carried out thoroughly and correctly, hand washing is the single most effective way to prevent the spread of infection.

1. Palm to palm.
2. Right hand over left dorsum and left palm over right dorsum.
3. Palm to palm fingers interlaced.
4. Backs of fingers to opposing palms with fingers interlocked.
5. Rotational rubbing of right thumb clasped in left palm and vice versa.
6. Rotational rubbing, backwards and forwards with clasped fingers of right hand in left palm and vice versa.

Note: Do not forget to include wrists and dry well, using disposable paper towels.

16.7.1   When you need to wash hands

- Before starting work and after leaving the work area.
- Before and after each contact with the service users.
- After handling used laundry and clinical waste.
- After contact with bodily fluids.
- After removing disposable gloves.

- Before and after handling and eating food.
- After using the toilet.
- After touching or blowing your nose.

16.8   Universal infection control precautions

The most important thing for a social care worker to do is to take steps to prevent infections by following the strict rules of universal infection control precautions. The term 'universal precautions' means undertaking safe working routine practices, to protect you and the service users from infection by blood and body fluids. Many diseases can be transmitted by infected blood or body fluids such as Hepatitis B, HIV and many others. Universal infection control precautions include:

- washing hands thoroughly with soap and running water (hot water);
- wearing disposable gloves;
- covering your mouth and nose, when sneezing, e.g. sneezes into a handkerchief or tissue if suffering from a cold;
- wearing protective clothes;
- disposing of waste properly.

16.9   General safety advice

- *Always* cover any open wounds with a dressing or a waterproof plaster. Uncovered open wounds are subject to invasion by viruses, which could possibly enter into the bloodstream. All bodily fluids are potentially dangerous, especially when near open wounds.
- *Always* wear gloves and aprons when cleaning up spills from bodily fluids or excreta. Wash blood splashes off skin immediately with running water.
- *Always* wash your hands after you have finished each task and wash your hands before leaving the service user or finishing a specific care task.
- *Never* transfer the same pair of gloves from one service user to another: it may cause cross contamination. Use a new pair of gloves with each task.
- *Cool* burn injuries as quickly as possible by immersing the affected area in cold water or applying ice packs. Apply a sterile, dry dressing avoiding any constriction of the area. Do not apply any creams or ointments or lotions unless under medical advice. Do not prick any blisters.
- *Always* wear sensible shoes at work.
- *Always* wear sensible clothes at work.
- *Remove* all facial piercings whilst at work with the exception of small studs or similar and appropriate earrings to the ear lobe.
- There are lots of ways to ensure safety. Start by learning what hazards you may face for each part of your job. Then find out what steps you and your service users should take to stay safe and prevent accidents.

16.10 Body fluids procedures

16.10.1 Introduction

Body fluid spills include blood, faeces, urine, vomit, tears, sweat, semen and anything else that comes from the person's body. Body fluid spills are a potential slip hazard. They may also potentially carry blood-borne viruses such as Hepatitis B & C and HIV, or other infections. Care must be taken when cleaning body fluid spills – always use a body fluid kit.

16.10.2 Body fluid kit

The body fluid kit is labelled 'biohazard kit' and should be located in the main offices of the services or in COSSHI storage areas. The body fluid kit contains the following:

- a yellow coloured mop and bucket;
- disposable plastic aprons;
- disposable cloths;
- eye protectors;
- container of bactericidal cleaning liquid;
- disposable plastic gloves;
- yellow clinical wastage sacks.

It is important to restock the kit after use and ensure that items remain in good condition.

16.10.3 Cleaning body fluid spills

- Body fluid spill should be dealt with promptly. Where possible, the area should be blocked off and other people should be warned of the hazard to keep them away.
- Always wear plastic gloves and aprons and ensure that they are in good condition, i.e. gloves have no tears. Over boots (on shoes) and face mask should also be worn – personal protective equipment as stipulated in the Health and Safety at Work Act – The Personal Protective Equipment Regulations 1992. Failure to do so will be at staff members' own risk.
- Never reuse gloves or other personal protective equipment.
- Be aware that fluids may be present on other surfaces such as door handles, clothing, beddings and walls. Extra care must be taken if other objects such as sharps are also present.
- Always cover cuts and grazes with water proof dressings. Do not attempt to clear spills if you have eczema or chapped skin.
- Use bactericidal cleaning liquid by spraying on the spills and use paper towels to remove as much materials as possible. Spray the bactericidal liquid again and clean with hot water. Carpets should be shampooed where required.
- In order to avoid contaminating other surfaces when removing waste whilst wearing gloves, where necessary obtain help in opening doors.
- Dispose of all waste materials (other than sharps) and protective equipment in yellow clinical waste sacks and keep separate from other waste. Follow the procedures laid down by your organisation on clinical waste disposal.

16.10.4 Contact with body fluids

Whilst cleaning the spill, if you come into direct contact with body fluids wash the affected area immediately with antibacterial soap and seek medical advice straight away especially if you have cuts or open wound or chapped skin.

16.11 Learning outcomes

- To understand the basic means and your role in infection prevention and control. For example this can include relevant contact numbers, the role of occupational health, and also:

  o safe use and disposal of sharps and management of accidental splash or sharps injuries;
  o management of blood and body fluid spillages;
  o maintenance of environmental cleanliness and impact on infection control.

- To understand the role of hand washing in the prevention of transmission of infection.
- To develop an understanding of the general principles of standard precautions.
- To outline how service users and visitors can contribute to infection prevention and control.
- To outline factors which may increase an individual's susceptibility to infection.
- To understand where additional information about infection prevention and control, including relevant national legislation or guidance and local policies, may be found/sought.

16.12 Framework for reflective practice

➤ *Knowledge:* What have you learnt from reading this chapter?
➤ *Skills:* What do you know, or can do differently now, that you did not/could not do before reading this chapter?
➤ *Practices:* How can you perform a task now better than before?

16.13 References

Ayliffe, G.A.J., Fraise, A.P. and Mitchell, K. (2000) *Control of Hospital Infection: A Practical Handbook*, 4th edn. London: Arnold.
Damani, N.N. (2003) *Manual of infection control procedures*, 2nd edn. London: Greenwich Medical Media Ltd.
Department of Health (1984) *Infection – Its Causes and Spread (Introduction). Public Health (Control of Disease) Act.* London: HMSO.
Department of Health (1998) *Guidance for Clinical Health Care Workers: Protection against Infection with Blood Borne Viruses.* London: DoH.
Department of Health (2006) *Infection Control Guidance for Care Homes.* London: DoH.
Health and Safety at Work Act 1974. London, HMSO

Health and Safety Commission (1992) *The Management of Health and Safety at Work Regulations.* London, HMSO.

Health and Safety Commission (1994) *A Guide to the Health and Safety at Work Act 1974.* Sudbury: HSE.

Horton, R. and Parker, L. (2002) *Informed Infection Control Practice (2nd ed.),* London, Churchill Livingstone.

HSE (1992) *Personal Protective Equipment Regulations 1992.* London: Stationery Office.

HSE (1999) *Control of Substances Hazardous to Health Regulations 1999.* London: Stationery Office.

Infection Control Nurse Association (2002) *Hand Decontamination Guidelines.* Huntington: ICNA.

Lawrence, J. and May, D. (2003) *Infection Control in the Community.* Scotland: Churchill Livingstone.

Wilson J. (2001) *Infection Control in Clinical Practice* (2nd ed.) Balliere Tindall, London

Woodburn, K. and Mackenzie, A. (2004) *Too Posh to Wash: The Complete Guide to Cleaning Up Your Life.* London: Michael Joseph.

16.14 Induction workbook

1. What are the main routes by which infection can enter the body?

_____

_____

2. Explain the universal infection control precautions.

_____

_____

3. How might your own health and hygiene pose a risk to service users?

_____

_____

4. Identify different types of personal and protective equipment (PPE) at the workplace and when to use each.

_____

_____

5. Why would you still need to wear personal protective equipment, even when you felt the risk of infection was minimal?

_____

_____

17   Food Handling and Hygiene

AIMS
- To be able to identify the potential where food hazards might occur
- To understand what cross-contamination is and how to avoid it
- To recognise ways of keeping food safe
- To understand how to store food – cooked and raw and high-risk foods
- To understand food poisoning causes and how to keep food safe

17.1   What is food hygiene?

Food hygiene is a way of keeping food safe for consumption. In the case of care environment this means handling and keeping food safe for consumption by service users, residents and colleagues. The handling of food and food hygiene is regulated by the following legislation:

- Food Safety Act 1990: This legislation sets out the requirements of the food producer and handler with respect to food safety.
- Food Hygiene (England) Regulations 2006.

All food preparation must be undertaken in accordance with the principles of Hazard Analysis and Critical Control Points (HACCP), i.e. ensuring food safety at all times. Further specific advice on food safety can be obtained by contacting your local environmental health department.

- The Health Act – 'Hygiene Code' 2006
- Food Hygiene (Eng) Regulations 2006
- Food Hygiene (EC) Regulations 852/2004
- The Food Safety Act 1990
- The Food Hygiene (General) Regulations 1970
- The Food Hygiene (Amendment) Regulations 1990
- The Health and Safety at Work Act 1974.

17.2   HACCP – Hazard Analysis Critical Control Point

HACCP is a tool used to minimise food hazards in food preparation in hospitals, care homes and all other catering operations. Food hazards can be identified and controlled in the following ways:

- Analyse potential food hazards.
- Identify the potential where food hazards may occur.
- Decide which points are critical to ensure safe food.
- Implement effective controls and monitoring.
- Review periodically.

In residential setting or projects where food is prepared for a large clientele, the critical control points on the hazard analysis sheets should be monitored by the person on cooking duty, recorded on the preparation and cooking record sheets, dated and signed.

17.3   General guidelines on food hygiene

17.3.1   Introduction

The harmful bacteria that cause food poisoning can spread very easily which can lead to serious illnesses or even death.

17.3.2   Who is at risk?

Some people are more vulnerable to food poisoning than others. This is particularly so among the high-risk groups such as children, pregnant mothers, and the elderly or immune-compromised people and allergy sufferers or people with illness. Therefore, good food hygiene is essential to ensure that any food stored or provided is safe.

17.3.3   Further guidelines

- Staff and service users engaged in the catering process should at all times maintain the highest standards of personal hygiene and cleanliness consistent with Environmental Health recommendations.
- Staff should encourage service users to assist in the kitchen subject to appropriate supervision and hygiene – washing hands before and after handling food.
- Any person working in the food area who knows or suspect that they are suffering from, or carriers of, any illness or condition likely to result in food contamination by micro pathogenis micro-organisms must advise the project or care setting manager as soon as possible.
- No persons who are known or suspected of suffering from, or the carrier of, any disease likely to be transmitted through food (e.g. by infected wounds and cuts, skin infections diarrhoea or sores) will be allowed to work in any food handling area or cook for service users, if there is a possibility of contaminating the food.

17.4   Cross-contamination and food poisoning

Contamination is the presence of any harmful substance or object in food (food hazards). This could be:
- food poisoning bacteria, viruses;
- physical objects like hair, wires, jewellery;
- chemicals – cleaning chemicals.

Cross-contamination is the transfer of bacteria from raw foods to other foods which can be done directly or indirectly (for example by hands, utensils, surfaces, cloths among others).

17.4.1   Some measures to combat cross-contamination

- Keep the raw food away from the ready to eat foods.
- Use different surfaces or chopping boards for different types of food, e.g. red board for raw meat, brown board for vegetables; green board for salads and fruits; blue board for raw fish; white board for bakery and dairy; yellow board for cooked meat.
- Store raw meat in sealable containers at the bottom of the fridge so it doesn't touch or drip onto other foods.
- Wash hands after handling food, especially raw meat.
- Wash knives/utensils thoroughly with hot water – where possible use separate equipment/utensils for raw food and ready to eat food.

17.4.2   Personal hygiene

Food can be easily contaminated when handling. Good standards of personal hygiene should therefore be maintained at all times by:

- washing and drying hands thoroughly and regularly, especially before starting work, before handling ready-to-eat foods, after handling raw meat, after breaks – smoking and using the toilet;
- avoiding sneezing/coughing over food;
- covering cuts and wounds with clean waterproof dressing;
- wearing clean clothes and protective garments like apron, hat and gloves (preferably blue as there is hardly any food that is coloured blue);
- not touching your hair, face or pick your nose when handling food.

17.4.3   Causes of food poisoning

Food poisoning is an acute illness usually occurring within 36 hours of consuming contaminated or poisonous food. Symptoms may last up to seven days and include:

- diarrhoea
- vomiting
- fever
- malaise
- abdominal pain
- loss of appetite.

Food poisoning can be caused by:

- germs in food
- bacterial/toxins
- chemicals in food
- metals in food
- viruses
- poisonous plants
- reactions

- poisonous fish.

Contamination can get into food in a number of ways:

- from raw food
- from dirty work surfaces
- from pets
- from packaging
- from equipment
- from cleaning products
- from you and your hands.

17.4.4 Causes of food poisoning outbreaks

Key factors involved in food poisoning outbreaks:

- preparing food too far in advance;
- contamination of processed food;
- storage at incorrect temperature, incorrect cooling, reheating or thawing;
- cross-contamination;
- infected food handlers;
- management failure.

17.4.5 Movement of bacteria

Bacteria need four things to grow; Food, moisture, water and time. Most bacteria can multiply by dividing themselves into two every 10–20 minutes (one bacteria can develop into two million after 7 hours). Bacteria have limited self-movement capacities; they require a vehicle to be transported and transferred to the food from the source: these include:

- chopping boards
- hands
- knives
- hand/food contact surfaces.

To prevent bacteria from growing:

- kill them with heat;
- stop them growing with cold;
- kill them with chemicals.

Beware: food may look, smell and taste normal even when it can cause food poisoning. Safe food preparation, handling and storage in domestic and work environment will protect you and the service users from food poisoning.

17.5   Temperature controls

Temperature controls are essential to keeping certain foods safe. Certain foods if they are not kept chilled or hot prior to serving toxins can form in the food.

- Food being kept hot should remain above 63 °C (145 °F).

- Foods that need to be chilled should be kept at 8 °C (46 °F) or below.
- Ensure probe thermometers where used are kept clean and disinfected occasionally and records of food probing are kept.
- Don't overstock the fridge – this will affect the circulation of cool air.
- Check and record fridge temperatures regularly to ensure they are working correctly and keeping food at the correct temperatures.
- Have fridge thermometers in place, it is a good practice.

17.6   Food preparation and cooking

When preparing food the following are some of the guidelines to help ensure food safety:

- Observe good personal hygiene – wash hands regularly.
- Clean and sanitise equipment and surfaces thoroughly before and after use.
- Use different chopping boards/surfaces for raw food especially meat and ready to eat foods.
- Wash all fruits, vegetables and salads foods if being served raw.
- Keep all chilled foods and goods out of the fridge for the shortest time possible.
- Where possible use different equipment/utensils for raw foods and ready to eat foods.
- Avoid unnecessary handling of food.

Note:
- The proper cooking of food ensures that food poisoning causing bacteria are killed.
- Reheated food should be piping hot throughout and should not be reheated more than once.
- Avoid putting foods into the fridge when still hot – they may warm up other foods being stored.

17.6.1   Cooling

Any cooked food which is to be served cold, such as boiled beef, must be removed from the cooking dish as soon as cooking is completed and placed in a clean cold dish, covered and place in a well ventilated area to cool so that it may be placed in the refrigerator within two hours of cooling.

17.6.2   Serving

All hot foods must be served immediately at temperatures above 63 °C. Meals that are left over after a period of one hour should be cooled, covered and kept in the refrigerator until needed. They should be labelled with the date when cooked and expected date of usage.

17.6.3   Reheating and use of over production (leftovers)

- All foods must be used within three days of cooking, i.e. it is cooked one day, used the next day, and if not used all items should be thrown away on the third day.

- All foods must be reheated to above 75 °C and this temperature must be recorded on the kitchen cooking record sheet, dated and signed.

17.6.4 Menu planning

These should take into consideration:

- the need to provide a well-balanced diet;
- service users' choice;
- provision of alternative meals to cater for specific service users' dietary, medical and religious needs or preference for vegetarian food;
- project managers and key workers should review and ensure food provision costs are monitored with the agreed individual's budget.

17.7   Food handling and storage

To ensure safe food handling, good hygiene practice should be followed at every stage, from receiving foods to serving of food by:

- keeping raw foods away from the ready-to-eat foods;
- storing dried foods off the floor, ideally in sealable containers, to protect from pests and contamination;
- never using food after the 'use by' date;
- observing temperature controls;
- following storage instructions on packaging and handling/labelling;
- checking deliveries are at the correct temperatures and that the food is not damaged (packaging/containers);
- using reputable suppliers whose supplies and sources can be easily traced back.

17.7.1 Storage

- The temperature of all refrigerators should be:

  o   kept at 5 °C;
  o   freezers at -20 °C;
  o   checked twice daily by the staff on duty;
  o   recorded on the cold storage record sheet, dated and signed.
- All raw meats should be stored in a separate freezer or at the bottom of the refrigerator or freezer where it cannot come into contact with other foods.
- All foods should be covered and dated before being stored in the refrigerator.

17.8   Cleaning up

It is of great importance that all equipment and services that come into contact with food are kept clean and disinfected by:

- cleaning surfaces, equipment and floors frequently to avoid build up of waste and dirt;
- cleaning as you go along – put pills, onions, potatoes in the food waste container;
- keeping waste storage areas clean and disinfected with bins lids closed;
- ensuring the cleaning equipment itself is kept clean;
- not allowing food or other waste to build up in the food area;
- making arrangements for rubbish to be removed regularly.

17.9 Safe food handling policy

The policy is designed to ensure that all staff and service users engaged in the process of food production and preparation are:

- fully competent and able to operate safe working practices;
- compliant with relevant legislation, environmental health and recommended procedures;
- providing food of high and nutritional balance, reflecting the needs of the service users and within their respective budgets.

17.9.1 Food safety tips

- Keep meat, chicken and fish covered and refrigerated.
- Cook all meals thoroughly.
- Store cooked meats away from uncooked meats.
- Do not leave food uncovered – use foil or cling film.
- Do not use foods that are past their 'use by' dates.
- Keep all food containers tightly covered.
- Keep work surfaces clean.

17.10 Learning outcomes

- To demonstrate understanding and knowledge of safe guarding the health of service users with specific skills, techniques, methods and responsibilities in food handling and hygiene.
- To demonstrate understanding and knowledge of specific principles of cleaning and sanitising food establishments.
- To demonstrate understanding and knowledge of specific details and elements of pest control and prevention.
- To demonstrate understanding and knowledge of appropriate controls and for monitoring and maintaining food safety standards.

17.11 Framework for reflective practice

➢ *Knowledge:* What have you learnt from reading this chapter?
➢ *Skills:* What do you know, or can do differently now, that you did not/could not do before reading this chapter?
➢ *Practices:* How can you perform a task now better than before?

17.12 References

Food Hygiene (EC) Regulations 852/2004
Food Hygiene (Eng) Regulations 2006.
Food Hygiene (Amendment) Regulations 1990
Food Hygiene (General) Regulations 1970.
Food Safety Act 1990.
Health Act 2006: Hygiene Code.
Health and Safety at Work Act 1974
Sprenger, R.A. (2010) *The Food Safety Handbook (Level 2)*, 29th edn. Doncaster: Highfield
Sprenger RA (2003) *The Essentials of Food Hygiene: A Guide for Food Handlers.* Doncaster: Highfield

17.13 Induction workbook

1. List the main causes of food poisoning?

2. List the potential hazards to health and safety associated with food and its preparation.

3. Describe practices that promote safe food preparation and food hygiene.

4. Outline the main legislation that regulate food handling and how they can be applied to your work setting.

5. How would you empower a service user to engage in healthy eating, taking into consideration cultural differences?

6. How can you break the chain of infection?

7. What is one of the main actions that can control and eliminate infection in any setting and how can you promote it among the people you support?

PART V

THE EFFECT OF SERVICE SETTING
ON SERVICE USERS AND YOU

18   Protection from Abuse

AIMS

- To identify different types of abuse and the signs that abuse may be occurring
- To show what you must do if abuse is suspected or disclosed
- To provide an introduction to the concept of whistle blowing
- To create awareness about the various forms of abuse
- To provide a four-point approach to abuse awareness

Everyone has the right to live his or her life free from fear, violence or harm. All adults have the right to be protected from harm or abuse. Everyone has the right to an independent lifestyle and the right to make choices, some of which may involve a degree of risk.

(Department of Health, 2000)

18.1   Introduction

This chapter introduces the topic of protecting people with learning disabilities from abuse.

- It identifies different ways to stop and eliminate abuse of any form
- It considers when and why people with learning disabilities may be particularly vulnerable to abuse.
- It looks at what a care worker must do if abuse is suspected or disclosed, in line with organisations and national policies.

18.1.1   Definition of abuse

Abuse is a violation of an individual's human and civil rights by any other person or persons.
(Department of Health, 2000)

18.1.2   Who is at risk?

A vulnerable person – adult or child – is one who may be unable to take care of themselves; protect themselves from harm; or prevent themselves from being exploited.
Adults may be vulnerable because they:

- have a physical disability;
- have learning difficulties;
- have mental health problems;
- are old, frail or ill; or
- are sometimes unable to take care of themselves or protect themselves without help.

An adult may also be vulnerable because of a temporary illness or difficulty, e.g. homelessness.
Children may be vulnerable because they:

- have a physical disability;
- have learning difficulties;

- are too young
- are sometimes unable to take care of themselves or protect themselves without help;
- may have difficulty in making their wishes and feelings known and this may make them vulnerable to abuse.

This may also mean that they are not able to make their own decisions or choices.

18.1.3 Who is an abuser?

Any of the following could potentially be an abuser:

- a partner or relative or other household member;
- friends or neighbours;
- health or social care worker;
- carer (residential setting);
- another customer or service user;
- any other person with access to the abused person concerned.

18.2 Forms of abuse

There are three forms of abuse.

18.2.1 Deliberate abuse

Deliberate abuse is where the abuser knows that she or he is abusing. It is pre-planned and often systematic, e.g. when a staff member plans to physically hurt a service user.
Deliberate abuse can be in the form of:

- bullying
- physical restraint

18.2.2 Spontaneous abuse

Spontaneous abuse is an isolated incident without pre-meditation, for example when a carer becomes frustrated by a challenging service user and starts shouting at them.
Spontaneous abuse can be in form of:

- shouting;
- swearing;
- pushing the service user.

18.2.3 Unintentional abuse

Unintentional abuse is the abuse that arises through neglect or poor practice, or where there are inadequate resources to provide the proper care that is needed, for example, when a carer fails to provide access to appropriate toileting services, or when a service user has been given too much medication by an untrained carer.

Unintentional abuse can be in form of:

- poor record-keeping;
- ignoring the service user;
- failure to provide access to appropriate health services.

18.3 Types of abuse

There are six types of abuse:

1. physical abuse
2. neglect
3. emotional abuse / psychological abuse
4. sexual abuse
5. institutional abuse
6. financial abuse

and each of them can take any of the three forms discussed earlier in the chapter.

18.3.1 Physical abuse

Physical abuse is one of the most common types of abuse. It can take place in many ways: hitting, slapping, rough handling, inappropriate restraints or sanctions, excessive or inappropriate use of medication.

Indicators of physical abuse can be in form of physical or behavioural indicators.

1. *Physical indicators*

(a) Unexplained bruises, welts, lacerations and abrasions:
- on the face, lips, mouth;
- on torso, back, buttocks, thighs;
- lacerations in various stages of healing;
- reflecting shape of an article used, e.g. belt buckle;
- bite marks or fingernail marks, scratches.

(b) Unexplained burns:
- especially on soles buttocks, arms, or back;
- immersion burns;
- electric burns (iron);
- rope burns.

(c) Unexplained fractures
- to the skull, facial structure;
- fractures in various stages of healing;
- multiple or spiral fractures.

2. *Behavioural indicators*

- Reluctant to change clothes in front of others.
- Wary of adult contact.
- Difficult to contact.
- Apprehensive when other children cry.
- Crying/irritability.
- Frightened of formal and informal carers.
- Behavioural extremes – aggression, withdrawal, impulsiveness.
- Apathy.
- Depression.
- Poor peer relationships.
- Panic in response to pain.

18.3.2 Neglect

Neglect occurs when a service user is not provided with adequate care and attention and suffers harm or distress as a result. Neglect and acts of omission include ignoring medical or physical care needs; failure to provide access to appropriate health, social care or educational services; the withholding of the necessities of life, such as medication, food and drink and heating.

Indicators of neglect

1. Physical indicators
   - constant hunger;
   - failure to thrive or malnutrition;
   - poor hygiene which may result in health problems;
   - unattended physical problems or medical needs.

2. Behavioural indicators
   - stealing food;
   - constant fatigue, listlessness or falling asleep;
   - alcohol or drug abuse;
   - aggressive or inappropriate behaviour;
   - isolation from peer group.

18.3.3 Emotional/psychological abuse

This can be more difficult to define and measure, because of this, it is often more difficult to detect and identify. Most obviously it can be seen as cruelty or verbal insults, but it can include shouting and swearing at service users, or even spreading rumours, malicious gossip or withholding of duty of care.

Indicators of emotional/psychological abuse

- Extreme low self-esteem.

- Compliant, passive, withdrawn, tearful. aggressive or demanding behaviour.
- Depression.
- Constant high anxiety.
- Poor social and interpersonal skills.
- Delayed development, i.e. speech.
- Persistent habit disorder, e.g. rocking, biting.
- Self-destructive behaviour.

18.3.4 Sexual abuse

Sexual abuse is any contact or interaction (physical, visual, verbal or psychological) between a child/adolescent and an adult (or another adult) when the child/adolescent/adult is being used for the sexual stimulation of the perpetrator or any other person, and – in the case of adults – without the mutual consent of both parties.

- Sexual abuse in the care setting is where the service user is forced to take part in sexual activity without their consent.
- Any kind of sexual relationship between a staff and a service user is abusive, even if consent is given.
- However, sexual abuse can take more subtle ways and can occur when staff are administering personal care, or making comments related to someone's sexual orientation or gender identity.

Indicators of sexual abuse

- Unexplained difficulty walking.
- Bleeding or bruised genitals.
- Complaining of pain while urinating or having a bowel movement, or exhibiting symptoms of genital infections such as offensive odours, or symptoms of a sexually transmitted disease.
- Reluctant to be alone with a particular person.
- Sudden behaviour change.
- Engaging in persistent sexual play with friends, toys or pets.
- Having unexplained periods of panic, which may be flashbacks from the abuse.
- Regressing to behaviours too young for the stage of development they already achieved.
- Initiating sophisticated sexual behaviours.

18.3.5 Institutional abuse

Institutional abuse is the mistreatment of people brought about by poor or inadequate care or support or systematic poor practice that affects the whole care setting. It occurs when the individual's wishes and needs are sacrificed for the smooth running of a group, service or organisation.

This type of abuse can be rife in areas where there is a very rigid and long-standing routine ('We have always done it that way.') Or when tasks are carried out for the 'good' of the staff, rather than in the best interest of service users, e.g. bath times, weigh days in prison or residential homes.

Indicators of institutional abuse

- Treating adults like children.
- Arbitrary decision making by staff group, service or organisation.
- Strict, regimented or inflexible routines or schedules for daily activities such as meal times, bed/waking times, bathing/washing, going to the toilet.
- Lack of choice or options such as food and drink, dress, possessions, daily activities and social activities.
- Lack of privacy, dignity, choice or respect for people as individuals.
- Unsafe or unhygienic environment.
- Lack of provision for dress, diet or religious observance in accordance with an individual's belief or cultural background.
- Withdrawing people from individually valued community or family contact.

18.3.6 Financial abuse

Financial abuse can take many forms, from staff denying service user all access to funds, to making them solely responsible for all finances while handling money irresponsibly themselves. Or this is the attaining of money, possessions or property through cheating or deception.

Indicators of financial abuse

- Sudden withdrawal of money from bank accounts.
- Loss of financial documents.
- Person with a disability is accompanied by family, staff or others who appear to coax, or otherwise pressure, the individual into making transactions.
- Persons accompanying the individual speak for her/him, and do not allow the individual to speak or make decisions.
- Individual expresses concern that s/he does not have enough money for basic needs.
- Individual is confused about missing funds in accounts.
- Sudden increase in checking overdrafts.
- Unusually large cash withdrawals or transfers to other accounts from a joint bank account, without the individual's knowledge or consent.
- Individual cannot obtain checking or savings passbooks from person assisting with finances, or passbook/cheque book are frequently missing.
- Individual complains that furniture, jewellery, credit cards, or other items are missing.
- The individual complains about not having access to her/his own money.
- Caregiver charging personal expenses to the credit card of an individual.
- Caregiver spending the individual's money for his/her own use.
- Caregiver coercing an individual to pay for his/her own expenses.

18.4 Why does abuse happen?

- Inadequate training of carers.

- Lack of person-centred care planning or a ritualised care routine.
- Working in isolation.
- Continued over-demanding behaviour.
- Communication difficulties.
- Drug and alcohol abuse.
- Stress within a relationship.
- Lack of support and or services.
- Reversal of roles – abused becomes the abuser.
- Poorly supervised.

18.5   What can you do to stop abuse?

- You must always act.
- Know your organisation's procedure for reporting abuse.
- If you suspect abuse, inform your line manager immediately.
- Speak to a service user's social worker.
- In the event of criminal behaviour, inform the police.
- Always check that action has been taken.
- Do not try too much by yourself.
- Respect the wishes of the individual and be sensitive to their cultural background.
- *Do not* promise to keep secrets.
- If possible act with the knowledge of the service user. If this is not possible you must still take action.
- Be aware of the need to protect and not contaminate evidence.
- Information that will be required will include what you have been told, by whom, what you yourself have observed, dates, times, locations, names, etc. Do not embroider the facts.
- Document and record everything.

18.6   Strategies to prevent abuse

To be able to prevent abuse there are certain things we must consider before every contact, intervention or response with the service user. We should always ask ourselves 'Is this in the best interest of the service user?' Every staff member should be able to justify their answer to this question.

There are five levels which we have to be aware of to be able to prevent abuse:

(a) service user;
(b) yourself (staff, volunteer workers, caregivers etc.);
(c) environment;
(d) organisation;
(e) current legislation and guidance.

What do you need to consider in order to prevent a potentially abusive situation arising?

(a) Service user

In order to prevent a potentially abusive situation from arising in a care environment staff should consider the following about the service user:

- Is there a care plan in place?
- Do I know it?
- What is the service user's wishes and preference?
- What is the communication potential/style? Verbal or nonverbal?
- What is the service user's pattern of communication – oral, written, sign, symbols or objects? Am I (staff) able to understand them?
- Are behaviour support plans in place?
- What is the mental/physical state of the service user?
- What control measures are in place?
- Has intervention been risk assessed?
- What has worked before?
- Can I avoid the intervention?
- Have other tactics be tried such as de-escalation?

(b) Yourself (staff, volunteer workers etc.)

As a member of the care team, consider how you could prevent a potentially abusive situation from arising by bearing in mind the following;

- Do I know the organisation's policy and procedure on safeguarding?
- Do I know the care plan? Has it changed recently?
- Do I know the potential risks involved, and how can I avoid them?
- Am I trained to do this?
- Do I know how to access support?

(c) Environment

With the insight knowledge staff have on the service user and themselves, they should assess how they could contribute towards preventing abuse from arising by considering the following in regard to environment:

- Is the area safe for the service user, is it too hot/cold/noisy? Are lights too dim/bright etc?
- Are there any trip hazards, sharps, electricity, etc?
- Are there doors/windows; are these closed, in the toilets and bathrooms?
- Are doors locked? Can they ensure privacy and dignity?

(d) Organisation

As staff, they should be able to know what the management can do to help combat the threat of abuse. The management should ensure that the potential for abuse is recognised and that strategies are put in place by:

- ensuring care plans are in place;
- the risk assessments are carried out, reviewed and up-to-date;
- training is up-to-date; who is trained in what;

- running Criminal Records Bureau checks;
- the staffing level is adequate;
- ensure consent is obtained on issues of confidentiality where appropriate;
- the care setting is registered with the relevant body (usually Care Quality Commission – CQC).

(e) Current Legislation and Guidance

The organisation does not expect staff to know the content of all pieces of legislation; however, staff are expected to work within the organisation's policies and procedures.

The following legislation or guidance should be available in place to raise awareness to avoid abuse. Depending upon the area, the legislation and guidance include:

- The Children and Young Persons Act 2008
- Deprivation of Liberty Safeguards Act 2007
- Mental Health Act 2007
- Safeguarding Vulnerable Groups Act 2006
- The Care Standards Act 2000
- NHS & Community Care Act 1990
- Offences Against the Person Act 1861
- Domestic Violence and Matrimonial Proceedings Act 1976
- Race Relations Act 1976
- The Human Rights Act 1998
- Sexual Offences Act 2003
- The Disability Discrimination Act 2005

18.6.1 Ways to prevent abuse

There are different *ways* that can help stop or prevent abuse from occurring in any care environment. Prevention needs to take place in the context of person-centred support and personalisation, with individuals empowered to make choices and supported to manage risks.

- The most common prevention intervention for adults at risk include training and education of the adults at risks themselves and staff on abuse in order to help them to recognise and respond to abuse.
- Other approaches include identifying people at risk of abuse.
- Raising awareness, information, advice and advocacy, policies and procedures, community links, legislation and regulations, interagency collaboration and a general emphasis on promoting empowerment and choice.
- Education: this involves providing service users with knowledge about their rights, and teaching them skills to identify abuse, ask for help, and avoid being re-victimised.
- Staff and caregivers need information and support to help them care for service users in a positive and an empowering manner.
- Increase knowledge about service users' abuse and its impact throughout different stages of life.

18.7 Four-point approach to abuse awareness

There is a four-point approach to abuse awareness.

18.7.1 Prevention

We have identified the issues involved about how we can use our knowledge of the service user, ourselves as staff, the environment, the organisation and legislation to prevent abuse.

18.7.2 Identification

We have identified the possible indicators of abuse, which help us to identify the potential of abuse occurring.

18.7.3 Action

Where abuse is suspected it should be reported. This can be done through the organisation's whistle-blowing policy and local authorities alerter's guidance. Or in your care setting through:

- immediate line manager;
- service manager;
- service provider;
- other relevant bodies.

All reports of abuse must be taken seriously. Every report must be investigated. This should be done quickly, fairly, and in an open and transparent manner. The most important aspect is the protection of the vulnerable person. To achieve safety:

- the person who is accused may be suspended from duty;
- this is not a disciplinary action and no one should consider it as such;
- it does not mean the person is guilt.

18.7.4 Planning

It is important that we learn from every instance, and that control measures are put in place to prevent a recurrence. In this the way the four-point approach plan becomes a dynamic tool.

18.8 Whistle blowing

Whistle blower is an informant who exposes wrongdoing within an organisation in the hope of stopping it. Employees and workers who make a 'protected disclosure' are protected from being treated badly or being dismissed.

The key piece of whistle-blowing legislation is The Public Interest Disclosure Act 1998 (PIDA) which applies to almost all workers and employees who ordinarily work in Great Britain.

18.8.1 Role of an organisation in whistle-blowing policy

- Organisations should provide sufficient training to enable recognition of abuse and carers responsibilities.
- Staff have the responsibility to highlight poor practice.
- Organisations should ensure sufficient staff support and reassurance.
- The organisations should provide protection against reprisals.

18.9 Current legislation and guidance

- The Children and Young Persons Act 2008
  An Act to reform the law relating to children
- Deprivation of Liberty Safeguards Act 2007
  These safeguards focus on those in hospital or within care homes who for their own safety and in their own best interest need to be accommodated under the care and treatment regimes that may have the effect of depriving them their liberty, but who lack the capacity to consent.
- Mental Health Act 2007
  The Act states that everyone should be treated as able to make their own decisions until it is shown that they can't. MHA 2007 also aims to enable people to make their own decisions for as long as they are capable of doing so.
- Safeguarding Vulnerable Groups Act 2006
  Creating the Independent Safeguarding Authority, the Safeguarding Vulnerable Groups Act, which came into force in November 2006, heralds very significant changes in the way people who work with children or vulnerable adults are vetted.
- The Care Standards Act 2000
  An Act to establish a National Care Standards Commission.
- NHS & Community Care Act 1990
  An Act to make further provision about health authorities and other bodies constituted in accordance with the National Health Services.
- Offences Against the Person Act 1861
  This Act Outlines the Offences that a person can commit against a fellow person.

18.9.1 Organisations involved in safeguarding (prevention of abuse)

There are some key organisations/agencies that may need to be involved in safeguarding concerns (abuse). It should be the service manager or senior staff in the management who should decide who to contact and take action in doing so, or staff should know the procedure to follow. Below are some of those to contact.

- **Police**
  Staff in a care environment should know the procedures of contacting the police, if at any time the situation involves something which is against the law, or the service user or a witness is in danger, then the police should be contacted immediately or at the earliest opportunity. The person in charge of the service should initiate this contact. In such cases, the police will need to gather evidence.

- **Local Authorities Designated Officer (LADO)**
  All staff and volunteer workers should know that each local authority has a LADO who should be alerted to all cases in which it is alleged that a staff or volunteer who works with vulnerable people has behaved in a way that has harmed or may have harmed a vulnerable person, or has committed a criminal offence against a vulnerable person or their behaviour towards vulnerable people indicates she/he is unsuitable to work with vulnerable people.

- **Social care team**
  The local authority social care team should be notified of any safeguarding concerns about any vulnerable person/child, and if the vulnerable person/child has a social worker, they should be contacted. In cases of registered looked after children, the concerned team should be contacted as well.

- **Adult social care team**
  If the vulnerable person is an adult, the local social services office or named care manager should be notified. Each and every vulnerable adult in any setting has a care manager who oversees their well-being; from housing needs, benefits etc. the local authority safeguarding team will consider the referrals, and offer advice on what action should be taken in response.

Staff should document everything that has taken place in the service user's daily diary and highlight the information for other staff in the Communication Book, referring them to the service user's diary, incident/accident form and police reference numbers or any other authority that may have been contacted.

18.10 Recording observable body injuries

The physical injuries or unexplained bruises found on the body of a service user must be shade and labelled on a diagram called a 'body map'.

The size, shape and colouring should equally be noted, this may help determine when the injuries occurred.

18.11 Learning outcomes

In the case of vulnerable children

- To understand what constitutes child abuse.
- To know about local policies/procedures.
- To know what to do if there are concerns.
- To understand the importance of sharing information, how it can help and the dangers of not sharing information.

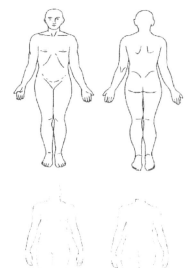

Figure 18.1 Body map

In the case of vulnerable adults

- To be aware of and be able to define 'vulnerable adult' as a term.
- To know about types of adult abuse and be able to recognise indicators of types of adult abuse and neglect. .
- To know about local arrangements for the implementation of multi-agency safeguarding adults policies and procedures.
- To know what to do if there are concerns.
- To understand the importance of sharing information, how it can help and the dangers of not sharing information.
- To know what to do if you experience barriers in alerting or referring to relevant agencies

18.12 Framework for reflective practice

➢ *Knowledge:*   What have you learnt from reading this chapter?
➢ *Skills:*   What do you know, or can do differently now, that you did not/could not do before reading this chapter?
➢ *Practices:*   How can you perform a task now better than before?

18.13 References

Amiel, S. and Heath, I. (eds) (2003) *Family Violence in Primary Care*. Oxford, Oxford University Press.
BILD (2010) Code of Practice for the Use and Reduction of Restrictive Physical Interventions. Kidderminster: BILD Publications.
Care Homes Regulations 2001, Private and Voluntary Health Care Regulations.
Children and Young Persons Act 2008.
Department for Education and Skills (2004) *Every Child Matters: Next Steps*. Nottingham: DfES.
Department for Education and Skills (2007) *Care Matters: Time for Change*. Nottingham: DfES.
Department of Health (2000) *No Secrets (Adult Protection)*. London: Home Office/ Department of Health
Safeguarding Vulnerable Groups Act 2006. Website at: www.opsi.gov.uk
Thompson, N. (2005) *Understanding Social Work: Preparing for Practice*, 2nd edn. London: Palgrave Macmillan.
Thompson, N. and Thompson, S. (2008) *The Social Work Companion*. London: Palgrave Macmillan.

18.14 Induction workbook

1. Abuse may occur in many types. Outline the different types of abuse.

   _____

   _____

2. Identify the signs and symptoms for each type of abuse.

   _____

   _____

3. Outline the factors that may make people with learning disabilities more vulnerable to abuse and neglect.

_____

_____

4. Explain how you can support people with learning disability to reduce their own vulnerability to abuse at your workplace.

_____

_____

5. Identify five situations and settings where people with learning disabilities may be particularly vulnerable to abuse.

_____

_____

6. Outline the key legislation and national policy that relate to protecting people with learning disabilities from abuse.

_____

_____

7. How can you record and document signs of suspected abuse in a service user?

_____

_____

19 Lone Working

AIMS
- To understand what lone working is and qualities required for a lone worker
- To understand forms violence can take
- To provide general guidelines for staff and service users' safety when working alone in a project or in the community
- To understand Health and Safety Guidelines on lone working
- To understand lone worker's responsibilities and personal safety
- To understand emergency recovery plan when lone working

19.1 Who is a lone worker and what is lone working?

Lone workers are defined by Health and Safety Executive as 'those people who work by themselves without close or direct supervision'. This may include those who work alone in specific areas or buildings such as supported living schemes, hostel, housing projects workers, key workers, single cover scheme workers, community floating support, tradespersons to name a few.

Lone working is covered by the Health and Safety at Work Act 1999 and the Management of Health and Safety at Work Regulations 1974. This legislation applies to all instances of lone working. Many organisations use the term 'lone worker' to describe an employee who normally works alone in a service or someone who provides support to clients in their own homes. They may be part of a team, but work on their own routinely and are not closely supervised. They may be office-based employees, Floating support workers working in the community. They may be permanent or agency employees in a service.

19.2 Qualities required for being a lone worker

Lone working or working alone for significant periods of time requires specific skills, experience or other qualities related to the job. These will include:

- the ability to manage a personal workload effectively;
- the ability to work unsupervised and using personal initiatives for periods of time;
- specific experiences for working with a particular service user group;
- good communication skills both verbal and written;
- particular competencies related to the job role, e.g. working in mental health services.

19.3 Health and safety guidelines

These guidelines are designed to work in conjunction with Health and Safety Executive (HSE) Guidance leaflet *Working Alone in Safety – Controlling the Risks of Solitary Work*, the National Lone Working and Working Alone Policy.

19.4   Legislation

There are two main pieces of legislation that will apply to lone working:

The Health and Safety at Work etc. Act 1974 (HASAWA) and the Management of Health and Safety at Work Regulations 1999.

- The Health and Safety at Work etc. Act 1974
  Section 2 sets out a duty of care on employers to ensure the health, safety and welfare of their employees whilst they are at work.

- The Management of Health and Safety at Work Regulations 1999: Regulation 3 states that every employer shall make a suitable and sufficient assessment of:
  o   the risks to the health and safety of his employees to which they are exposed whilst they are at work; and
  o   the risks to the health and safety of persons not in his employment arising out of or in connection with the conduct by him of his undertaking

19.5   Responsibilities of employers

The Health and Safety at Work Act 1974 and the Management of Health and Safety at Work Regulations 1999 (as amended) place the duty of care on employers to ensure as far as is reasonably practical that:

- employees who are required to work alone or unaccompanied for significant periods of time are protected from risk to their health and safety;
- the risk to employees' health and safety are identified by risk assessment of the environment and where necessary, introduce measures to reduce any risk to an acceptable level by installing CCTV, personal alarms;
- employees are to raise an alarm when required;
- employees are adequately trained, with formal training wherever possible, prior to being expected to undertake lone worker duties;
- lone worker should be given information to deal with normal everyday situations but also understand when and where to seek guidance from others in unusual or threatening situations;
- an adequate handover system should be in place to enable relevant information to be passed on to safeguard the lone worker, e.g. information on the nature of clientele in a project/a home;
- all lone worker equipment are fully operational and occasioned spot checks are undertaken on personal alarms and mobile phones;
- any implementation of any reasonable changes to the lone worker's job or conditions for safety reasons should be identified during supervision and where necessary such changes should be acted upon and communicated to the lone worker;
- they can undertake, through their line managers, regular assessment of the risks lone workers may face at least annually or at times when there has been a change in

circumstances; for example increased level of physical violence against staff from service users.

19.6　Lone worker responsibilities and personal safety

The Health and Safety at Work Act 1974 also places a duty of care on employees to take reasonable care for their own safety and that of anybody affected by their actions or omissions.
Employees must also:

- follow the safety procedures set down at work;
- report any shortcomings or failings in the safety procedures to the project manager or supervisor or team leader;
- report any incidents of violence or aggression and near misses; these should include where a situation could have resulted in actual violence;
- take reasonable and practical measures to ensure their personal safety by carrying on themselves equipment that is fully operational like personal alarms, fully charged mobile phones and torches during building checks at night etc.

Before a staff member arranges a visit to lone work in the community, they may find it essential to consider the following:

- Do they really need to make this visit and do they need to go alone? Could the service user come to the office?
- Have they left details of the whereabouts on the information board and with their colleagues?
- Have they undertaken their own personal safety checks?
- Is their mobile phone charged and does it have calling credit?
- Do they feel confident to undertake the visit on their own?
- Are they content with the safety measures in place?

When female staff become pregnant, it's their responsibility to notify their employer immediately for a risk assessment to determine whether lone worker element of their duties should be continued.

19.7　General guidelines for staff and service users' safety when working alone

- All lone workers should be inducted thoroughly and receive a full handover before commencing their shift.
- They should be given information to deal with normal everyday situations but should also understand when and where to seek guidance from others in unusual or threatening situations like calling the police.
- All lone workers should have had a full Criminal Records Bureau check before commencing lone working for any care setting.

- All lone workers should read, sign and understand the professional boundaries and protection from abuse policies. This knowledge should be updated regularly.

In accordance with these policies of professional boundaries:

- lone workers are not permitted to act inappropriately towards the service users;
- lone worker should not make physical contact with the service users;
- lone workers should not say anything inappropriate to any service users at any time.

Lone workers should have regular reviews with the line manager in their working organisations to ensure their knowledge of lone working policy is up to date and appropriate for continued lone working.

19.8   Call in/out procedure

- Lone worker should make sure that they use the lone working forms to record staff from sister projects or log in with the response team at the start and end of each shift stating where they are working, start and expected finish times.
- If staff at sister project are lone working and call in when you are on your shift, record what time their shift starts and is expected to finish and their location.
- Persistent failure to use the call in/out procedure may result in breach of lone working procedure.
- As a lone worker staff should be aware of their personal safety and the potential risks. They should ensure they are familiar with the layout of the buildings, keep a direct exit route available and avoid situations that may lead to increased risk.
- If as a lone worker, staff feel threatened or at risk they should stay locked in the office and call the police (999). They should not leave the office, unless staying locked up in the office would be more dangerous to their health and safety or the health and safety of others.
- If as a lone worker, staff feel at risk to their personal safety and the project is unmanageable, they should alert the police by calling 999, or pressing the panic alarm that are linked to the police stations. They should inform and liaise with the on-call manager for support and guidance. They should lock the office and leave, taking with them the project/home mobile phone, and leaving a note on the office door with the office mobile number and stating where they have gone.
- In case staff cannot leave the project/home due to the presence of vulnerable people at site, call 999 and offer reassurance till help arrives; in case of fire staff should leave the building and summon help from outside. Staff safety comes first.
- Staff should liaise with the police to ensure the safety and security of service users and the building, and return to the project when measures are in place to appropriately manage the risk.
- As a lone worker, staff should at all times carry a portable (mobile) phone, whether one provided by the project or their own. (In most cases, projects/homes provide a mobile phone as additional equipment for safety.)

- Do not enter a service user's room alone unless not doing so would be detrimental to the safety of staff, the service user or the building.
- When lone working in high-risk projects, the management always devises a puzzle word to alert the police or fellow staff that staff are in danger without alarming the person who is causing the threat.
- If staff or other visitors are in danger, staff must use a password or sentence to alert their colleagues or the police. For instance, 'I think I've left the safe unlocked' or 'I have left the red diary on the desk.' This should get staff help as soon as possible.
- As a lone worker, staff should never hesitate to call the police when concerned about their safety or if they are a victim of a violent incident.

19.9   Lone working with a service user at a project, with other staff in another part of the building

- Staff should let the other member they are working with know where they are and what they are doing, where they are going and how long they would be.
- The staff in the main office should check up on their colleague if they are not back when expected.
- Staff should always carry a mobile phone when lone working anywhere on the project.
- Staff should not lone work with a service user when they are under the influence of alcohol or drugs.
- If a service user has a history of violence and or aggression, do not lone work with them unless it would be detrimental to their health not to do so.
- If staff feel uncomfortable working with a service user at any time, they should return to the office and lock the door, or if they were working in the office look for an excuse to leave the office, requesting the service user to leave as well.

19.10   Lone working with service users in the community

It is of paramount importance before staff set out to work with service users in the community to:

- Obtain all information they can about the service user first. This should allow them to manage any potential problems and put appropriate management in place. If there is a history of violence or aggressive behaviour, then risk assessment must be done for that specific service user and the purpose of staff lone working in the community, and possibly an additional member of staff should have to accompany them.
- Staff to ensure that they are familiar with the location of where they are going, and if they are going to visit a potential move-on property with a service user they should try and arrange for a member of staff from the corresponding company or organisation to meet them there.
- Never take any money from service users when lone working with them away from the project, for any reason whatsoever.
- If staff suspects the service user is under the influence of alcohol or drugs, they should not go with them but reschedule the event for a later date.

- Members of staff are not permitted to get in a car, their own or anyone else's, with a service user. Where transport is necessary, they should use public transport. In case of a medical emergency, call for an ambulance and police.
- Staff should always take what is essential with them for their lone working session. They should not take any items with them which they would not want the service user to read.
- Staff should always feel free to leave in the middle of a session if they feel at risk at any time and return to the project and inform their response team of their decision to terminate the session.
- Staff should always carry a mobile phone with them and a personal alarm that they can easily access.
- Staff should always tell a colleague where they are going, when their expected time of return is.
- Staff should also call the office every hour to check in.
- In most projects there is usually an out of office information board for check in/out. Staff should make sure they update the board when leaving the office and call in when they are expected

19.11 Lone working in an emergency situation

- If lone working in the community staff should try to get to a place of safety walking along places with CCTV, or at least a public place. Then they should use the mobile phone to call the project or the police if necessary.
- If staff feel at risk, and cannot get to a safe place or a public place, they should call the project and inform them where they are using the password or the sentence 'I think I've left the safe open' or whatever the password for their project is. This will alert their colleagues that they feel they are in danger and the colleagues will act upon message and call 999, alert the police as to where they are and other details of the situation that they know.
- If lone working on the project with another member of staff in another area of the project, return to the office and lock the door if it's safe to do so and if possible call the other member of staff to return to the office and if necessary call the police to attend if staff feel unsafe.

19.11.1 Emergency recovery plan when lone working

Every organisation must have their own emergency procedures in place, which describe what to do in the event that someone does not check in or calls for help in an emergency or in event of a crisis. If a lone worker has not checked in or come back at the time they had stated:

- The first thing to do is call the mobile phone number they are carrying, and if there is no response call their personal mobile phone and leave a message, as they may just have forgotten to check in.
- Wait for a certain length of time – this should be dependent upon agreement of what is appropriate for different situations. In some circumstances staff should not wait at all but proceed straight away to emergency procedures.
- If there is no response, staff should advise the project manager or other colleagues.

- Establish their last expected location and if possible try to contact that place.
- If concern is high, police should be contacted and arrange an immediate police visit to their last known location.

19.12 Personal lone worker safety checks

The safety checks lone workers should undertake are as follows.

19.12.1 Task

- Have there been changes to the task staff originally intended to do?
- Is the task likely to generate a hostile reaction from the service user?
- Is the task physically, mentally or emotionally challenging?

19.12.2 Time

- Is it a higher risk time of day/night?
- What has happened recently that might affect the current task?

19.12.3 Equipment

Have staff got all the equipment they need to deal with a safety situation/emergency?

- Working phone/personal alarm.
- Identification card.
- Emergency phone numbers and check in details.
- Small amount of money for a taxi in case of need to get away fast.
- Other items identified in the lone working risk assessment?

19.12.4 Place

- Do staff know where the entrances and emergency exits are and can they be easily accessed?
- Are there animals or other potential hazards? Dogs, snakes, hamster?
- What is the general condition of the environment – slip/trip hazards, cleanliness, poor lighting etc?
- If out of office, can staff get to and from the venue safely?
- Is there a good phone reception network?

19.12.5 People

- How skilled and confident are staff in their abilities to deal with task?
- Are there unexpected visitors/people there with the service user?
- Does the service user or anyone of the visitor appear to be under the influence of alcohol or drugs? Sign of empty beer cans, strong smell of cannabis etc.?
- Does the service user appear distressed, anxious, or angry to the point where staff have concerns for their safety? Screaming or shouting?

- Is anyone known to have or appear to have, an infectious disease? Like chicken pox?

19.12.6 Mobile phones

- Mobile phones must be kept fully charged and any technical faults should be reported immediately.
- In high-risk environment a lone worker should enter a message seeking emergency assistance, into auto text facility of the mobile which is linked to the response team. It would be easier to send an automated text message rather than try to telephone for assistance manually.
- The mobile phone should never be left unattended. It should be kept close at hand in case a situation arises.
- Lone workers could unintentionally increase the risk of aggression by using a mobile phone. In these circumstances you should use the mobile phone in a sensitive and sensible way.
- With lots of complicated new mobile handsets, lone workers should familiarise themselves on how to use their mobile telephones, although it should not be the only source of communication to their emergency contact telephone number.
- Before undertaking a visit, the signal level should be checked and if it is insufficient staff should contact their response team and let them know they are starting lone working, giving the location and the estimated duration of the visit. Once the visit has been completed the staff should notify the response team or the office.

19.12.7 Personal alarms

- As a lone worker staff should ensure their personal alarm is working.
- The personal alarms should be tested regularly to ensure operational equipment is in use.
- As a lone worker, staff should ensure their personal alarm is either carried in their hand, or alternatively it is placed in a readily accessible pocket or clipped onto a belt. It should not be concealed in a bag or briefcase. When triggered, the alarm should be pointed at the aggressor and then thrown so as to divert their attention to silencing the alarm, thus providing an opportunity for staff to get out of the environment and seek help.
- When an emergency or false alarm has been raised, the response team or project manager should review how the incident was handled and whether the current procedures require amending. 'Your safety is your priority.'

19.13 Lone working in a service user's home

19.13.1 Responsibility of employers

According to Health and Safety Executive employers of lone workers should:

- involve staff or their representatives when undertaking the required risk assessment process;
- take steps to check control measures are in place (examples of control measures include instructions, training, supervision and issuing protective equipment);

- review risk assessment annually or, as few workplaces stay the same, when there has been a significant change in working practice; when a risk assessment shows it is not possible for the work to be conducted safely by a lone worker, risks should be addressed by making arrangements to provide help or back-up;
- where a lone worker is working at another employer's workplace, that employer should inform the lone worker's employer (recruiting agency) of any risks and the required control measures.

19.13.2 Responsibility of staff

- Staff to respect the personal space of the service user they visit in their own homes.
- To take a flexible and responsive approach to the individual needs and wishes of each service user.
- To identify and promote best practice in supporting service user to enhance safe lone working.

When working in a service user's home, it is important to remember that staff are visitors and that they are entering the service user's private space and it must be respected as such.

19.13.3 Good values and principles for lone working in service user's house

1. *Acceptable behaviour from a lone worker*

- Calling before going over to announce their arrival time if it is not a shift working pattern.
- Knocking on the door and waiting to be invited in.
- Showing their identification and stating their business, e.g. link work.
- Asking to use facilities in the house such as:

  o to use the toilet;
  o to make a cup of tea/coffee;
  o to open the windows and curtains: for some service users it's part of their morning routine/ritual and should be considered as a possible trigger for anxiety or challenging behaviour.

2. *Behaviour unacceptable from a lone worker*

- Knocking on the door and walking in without being invited in.
- Not acknowledging the service user as staff walk into the house without greetings.
- Walking into the kitchen and helping themselves to tea/coffee without asking.
- Opening windows and curtains without asking.
- Using bathroom without asking.
- Not introducing themselves to the service user.

At the same time, when staff are working in a service user's home, it is their workplace and they remain responsible for their own health and safety. It is important, therefore, to maintain and reflect professional values and principles regarding working effectively with service users at all times.

19.13.4 Confidentiality and lone working

- Often working with a service user in their own home will mean working with them alone; however, other people may visit, e.g. social worker, relative or friends. As far as possible, information about other people who may be present when they visit should be clearly identified in the lone working risk assessment and a risk management put in place.
- If staff arrive for a visit for link work or advocacy and find unexpected visitors, they should assess whether or not they can safely and effectively work in that situation. If not, they should withdraw and arrange another time to meet with the service user.

19.13.5 Possible risks faced by a lone worker in a service user's home

Lone working is seen as the most appropriate and positive way of offering support to the service user. However, there are some possible risks:

- verbal/physical attack resulting in psychological harm to the worker;
- the worker could be verbally or physically attacked; for instance if the service user is under the influence of alcohol or they are distressed or angry to the point where they lash out blindly;
- a worker could have allergic reaction to pets;
- a worker could be bitten by a dog or scratched by a cat or pet hamster;
- unpredictable and possible violent reactions to a worker causing psychological or physical harm, especially when a task is likely to generate a hostile reaction from the service user.

19.14 Sharing information about risks with people outside the staff team

The risks lone workers face during the course of their work should be routinely assessed and kept under review as part of assessment and support planning. Staff should remain attentive to changing circumstances through their day-to-day work.

Where risks have been identified the need to share information with others will need to be considered. This may be necessary to ensure any agreed risks are supported and monitored by others as well as to keep others informed of potential risks the lone worker may face. Information about a service user may be passed to someone else:

- with the service user's consent;
- on a 'need to know' basis, because s/he will be involved in supporting the service user; for example where staff from more than one agency are involved, the service user needs to be told that some sharing of information is likely to be necessary – where appropriate;
- in some cases if the need to protect the public/others outweighs the duty of confidence of the service user.

Where risks of dangerous behaviour are identified, lone workers have absolute responsibility to take action with a view to reducing the risk and ensuring it is managed.

19.15 Learning outcomes

- To have an increased/renewed awareness of the personal safety issues concerning lone worker status.
- To be able to state they are aware of the strategies they can choose to adopt in relation to personal safety and the lone worker.
- To be able to state they are aware of the strategies that can be introduced by their organisation in relation to increasing the personal safety of alone workers.
- To be able to state that due to their increased/renewed awareness of personal safety issues arising from being a lone worker they are and feel safer performing their work.

19.16 Framework for reflective practice

- ➢ *Knowledge:*   What have you learnt from reading this chapter?
- ➢ *Skills:*   What do you know, or can do differently now, that you did not/could not do before reading this chapter?
- ➢ *Practices:*   How can you perform a task now better than before?

19.17 References

Bibby, P (1995) Personal Safety for Healthcare Workers. Aldershot: Ashgate.

Department of Health (2000) *NHS Zero Tolerance Campaign.* London: DoH.

Health and Safety at Work etc. Act 1974 (available at http://www.hse.gov.uk/legislation/hswa.htm).

Health Service Circular (2001) *Withholding Treatment from Violent and Abusive Patients in NHS Trusts,* HSC 2001/18.

HSE (1997) *Successful Health and Safety Management* HSG65, 2nd edn.

HSE (1997) *Violence and Aggression to Staff in Health Services, Guidance on Assessment & Management.* HSE Books

HSE (1999) *Health and Safety at Work etc. Act, 1974 – Guidance on the Act* (L1) HSE Books.

HSE (1999) *Management of Health and Safety at Work Regulations 1999* (http://www.hse.gov.uk/pubns/hsc13.pdf).

HSE (1999) *Management of Health & Safety at Work Regulations, 1999 Approved Code of Practice & Guidance* (L21). HSE Books

HSE (2006) *Violence to Staff.* IND (G) 69L8/92.

Management of Health and Safety at Work Regulations 1999.

NHS (2008) *Against Staff and Operates a Zero Tolerance Policy* (available at http://www.southstaffordshirepct.nhs.uk/policies).

NHS (2009) *Not Alone: A Guide for the Better Protection of Lone Workers in the NHS.* NHS CFSMS.

NHS (2010) *Incident and Near Miss Reporting and Management Policy* (available at http://www.porthosp.nhs.uk).

NHS (2010) *Policy and Guidelines for Dealing with Physical and Non-Physical Assaults* (available at http://www.southwestlondon.nhs.uk).

NHS Direct website. National Lone Working Policy.

Royal College of Nursing (1998) *Safer Working in the Community.* London: RCN.

19.18 Induction workbook

1. What difficulties are you likely to face when working alone?

   _____

   _____

2. What can you do to reduce or avoid these problems?

   _____

   _____

3. What are the responsibilities of an employer to a lone worker?

   _____

   _____

4. What are your responsibilities for your safety as a lone worker?

   _____

   _____

5. What precautions should you adhere to while lone working in the community?

   _____

   _____

6. What are the policies and procedures of lone working in an organisation's settings?

   _____

   _____

20 Violence at Work

AIMS
- To enable staff to appreciate the particular risks associated with lone working
- To ensure that safety precautions and emergency procedures are understood
- To assist staff to recognise and respond correctly to hazards arising during lone working

20.1 Introduction

This chapter deals with attacks upon staff or members of the public from service users.

- It is the responsibility of the organisation (employer) to recognise and maintain the health and safety of all employees and volunteers, and as such will take reasonable steps to prevent violence at work.
- The organisations should ensure the provision of safe working systems of work, suitable protective equipment and appropriate information for all staff and volunteers.
- Where incidents of violent behaviour occur, the victim should be provided with appropriate help and support like debriefing.

20.2 Definitions

The Department of Health has defined violence and aggression as 'any incident where staff are abused, threatened or assaulted in circumstances relating to their work, involving an explicit or implicit challenge to their safety, well-being or health'.

In accordance with the Health and Safety Executive, violence at work is defined as 'any incident in which a person is abused, threatened or assaulted in circumstances relating to their work'. Abuse on the other hand includes verbal abuse in all degrees or threats and counts just as much as a physical attack.

20.3 Types of violence at work

- shouting verbal/racial/sexual abuse
- pushing
- spitting
- objects thrown
- damage to property
- hostage situation
- locking staff in
- threats
- physical violence.

20.4 Legislation governing the management of violence at work

There are four main Acts from which regulations and orders arise.

- The Health and Safety at Work etc. Act 1974

Employers have a legal duty under this Act to ensure, so far as is reasonably practicable, the health, safety and welfare at work of their employees.

- The Management of Health and Safety at Work Regulations 1992
  Employers must assess the risks to employees and make arrangements for their health and safety by effective:
  o planning
  o organisation
  o control
  o monitoring and review.
  The risks covered should, where appropriate, include the need to protect employees from exposure to reasonably foreseeable violence.
- The Reporting of Diseases and Dangerous Occurrences Regulations (RIDDOR) 1995
  Employers must notify their enforcing authority in the event of an accident at work to any employee resulting in death, major injury or incapacity for normal work for three or more consecutive days. This includes any act of non-consensual physical violence done to a person at work.
- Safety Representatives and Safety Committees Regulations 1977(a) and The Health and Safety (Consultation with Employees) Regulations 1996(b)
  Employers must inform, and consult with, employees in good time on matters relating to their health and safety. Employee representatives, either appointed by recognised trade unions under (a) or elected under (b) may make representations to their employer on matters affecting the health and safety of those they represent.

20.5   Why violence occurs at work

Violence faced by staff in social and healthcare arises primarily because the work involves coming into contact with a wide range of people in circumstance which may be difficult. The service users and their relatives may be anxious and worried. Some service users may be predisposed towards violence. Risk of violence is increased in particular circumstances like:

- lone working;
- working after normal working hours;
- working with people who are emotionally or mentally unstable;
- working with people who are under the influence of drink or drugs;
- working with people under stress;
- working and travelling in the community;
- handling valuables or medication.

20.6   Responsibilities of staff

The Health and Safety Executive stipulates the responsibilities of staff as:

1. It is the duty of every staff member (agency workers included) to report any instance of violence (including verbal abuse) in the workplace on a serious incident report form. This should be done as soon as possible after the incident.
2. While attempting to prevent an act of violence no member of staff should risk their own safety, or the safety of others.

3. All staff have a responsibility not to endanger themselves or others. In particular they must not use provocative language or gestures towards service users.
4. Staff must take steps to familiarise themselves with the written policies and procedures which are provided by the organisations for safe systems of working, to ensure their safety at work at all times.
5. Staff subjected to violence will be entitled to take sick leave, support and access services including counselling and debriefing to prevent psychological trauma.
6. In an emergency member of staff should use the emergency services wherever possible by dialling 999 for police.
7. The senior worker on a project is authorised to take whatever immediate action is believed necessary in order to deal with any violent incident. For example, physical restraint if trained to do so.

20.7   Prevention

1. Risk assessments of areas and service users should be carried out in accordance with the Health and Safety Policy, which should be reviewed annually, or on every occasion when there is any change in procedures or substances that affects the risk, and when a violent incident has taken place.
2. Organisations recognise their responsibilities to take reasonable steps to significantly reduce the risk in all areas of work by carrying out thorough risk assessment of the project or residential care setting.
3. All staff should have training and information in identified risk areas within their place of work, and follow-up refresher courses and updated information as required.
4. Individual staff risk assessment should also be carried out for lone workers; these should be reviewed during the first six months and further information provided as follow up.
5. Should there be any outstanding actions identified by a risk assessment, actions should be taken as soon as is reasonably possible.

20.8   Reporting of violent incidents

- All violent incidents should be reported in accordance with serious incident policy.
- It is the responsibility of the project manager to report immediately if an incident occurs in their specific area, who will then review the existing risk assessment within a given duration of time e.g. five working days and any action identified should be taken as soon as is reasonably possible.
- All staff are required to report any incidents of violence, abuse or other incidents that concern them to their project managers or shift leader. These incidents, along with the information about the assailants, should be passed to help in reviewing the risk assessment.
- All information of reported incidents of violence should be shared as appropriate; especially information on individuals who pose repeated significant risk within the project should be passed to other organisations in accordance with the confidentiality policy.

20.9   Action and advice on dealing with aggression

- If any member of staff feels they are in danger they should, where possible, leave and summon help immediately.
- Staff should always make themselves aware of specific precautions to be taken in their workplace, e.g. wearing a personal alarm, keeping the exit route clear and in sight.
- Staff should never underestimate a threat or be drawn into an argument and never respond in an aggressive manner.
- Up to 90% of communication between individuals is nonverbal, so try to ensure you are not adopting body language that is aggressive, e.g. hands on your hips, or pointing fingers while addressing the service user.
- If you think you have done something to trigger the aggression, consider if you are the best person to deal with the situation or whether someone else could handle the situation more effectively (diffusion model).
- Be aware of the personal space (the length of your outstretched hand in front of yourself defines your personal space); keep your distance. Remember that everyone is different so allow an aggressor room to breathe.
- Staff should never put their hands on someone who is angry.
- Remember that many factors, e.g. stresses, frustrations, expectations, levels of learning disabilities, can influence how people react to situations, always be aware of as many of these factors as possible.
- Never turn your back on an aggressor, in case of physical attack get away to a place of safety as fast as you can.
- If you witness an aggressive situation think before you get involved. You may be more useful if you call for help.

20.10   Learning outcomes

To identify and understand:

- the context of personal safety in a lone working environment;
- health and safety implications of lone working management – safe systems of work;
- how to minimise the likelihood of an incident occurring in the community by detecting 'pre- incident indicators';
- how to recognise the cues prior to a person becoming very aggressive or violent;
- appropriate ways of using body language and subtle barrier signals to improve safety;
- verbal defuse strategies which de-escalate and reduce risk of violence;
- time, distance and opportunity in relation to exit/escape route proximity;
- the rights, responsibilities and implications of using force to disengage or defend oneself;
- how to use lone worker alert devices most effectively;
- own and others response to conflict, the support available and the importance of reporting.

20.11 Framework for reflective practice

- ➤ *Knowledge:*   What have you learnt from reading this chapter?
- ➤ *Skills:*   What do you know, or can do differently now, that you did not/could not do before reading this chapter?
- ➤ *Practices:*   How can you perform a task now better than before?

20.12 References

Department of Health (2001) *National Task Force on Violence Against Social Care Staff – Report and National Action Plan* [online].

Department of Health (2002) *NHS Health Development Agency: Violence and Aggression in General Practice: Guidance on Assessment and Management*. London: DoH.

Health and Safety at Work etc. Act 1974 (available at http://www.hse.gov.uk/legislation/hswa.htm).

HSE (1997) *Violence and Aggression to Staff in Health Services: Guidance on Assessment and Management*. HSE.

HSE (2011) Five Steps to Risk Assessment (available at www.hse.gov.uk/pubns/indg163.pdf).

Linsley, P. (2006) *Violence and Aggression in the Work Place: A Practical Guide for All Health Care Staff*. Abingdon: Radcliffe.

Management of Health and Safety at Work Regulations 1999. http://www.hse.gov.uk/pubns/hsc13.pdf

Rippon, T.J. (2000) Aggression and violence in health care professions, *Journal of Advanced Nursing* **31**(2): 452–60.

Shepherd, J. (1994*) Violence in Health Care: A Practical Guide to Coping with Violence and Caring for Victims*. Oxford: Oxford University Press.

20.13 Induction workbook

1. What are your responsibilities and the role of others in relationship to maintaining a safe environment?

    _____

    _____

2. Describe a situation that may be a risk to you. What do you understand in regard to the policy and practice of workplace about protecting yourself from violence?

    _____

    _____

3. List the security measures in the work place, for example locks, burglar alarms and identifying staff and visitors

    _____

    _____

4. What are the guidelines for staff working alone in case of a threatening situation like physical aggression?

    _____

    _____

5. Define and identify the measure to take when face with violence at work while lone working.

    _____

    _____

PART VI

DAILY PROCEDURES AND OPERATIONS

21 Communication Book: Handover and Ending the Shift Procedures

21.1 Guidelines for using the communication book

The communication book is a crucial tool in enabling effective communication within a shift-working staff team. It is a legal document and in order to ensure its proper and appropriate use, here are some guidelines which you should follow:

1. Indicate clearly the day and date at the start of each day, e.g. Monday, 25 June 2012.
2. Clearly identify who the message is intended for.
3. If there is a need to refer to the service user use *only* initials.
4. Anything referring to the service user's support should be recorded in their daily diaries, then a reference made in the communication book stating 'refer to the service user's daily dairy'.
5. Complaints should not be written in the communication book; this should be addressed verbally with the project/residential/ manager or follow the complaint procedure.
6. Any information of a confidential nature – for example, being unhappy about the action of an external organisation – should not be included in the communication book. Use a more professional method of raising the issue.
7. Be aware of how your message could be perceived; you may be annoyed that this is the fourth week the repairs have not been logged, but writing a message about it in large or capital letters may lead to the team members feeling harassed and justified in making a complaint. Messages should be accurate and non-discriminatory
8. The communication book is not the place to air grievances (see Grievances and complaints policy and procedures, Section 6.5).

21.2 Handover

1. When you start your shift, you should be given a handover, so that you know anything significant that has happened that day or since you last worked on the service (project or residential care setting) or if it's your first time at the service (project or residential care setting).
2. Please read the latest entries in the communication book for an update of what's been happening on the service.
3. Any significant conversations or events while you are on shift should be documented in the appropriate service user's daily diary, making a reference for staff to see the daily dairy in the communication book.
4. In residential care settings never leave the service user by themselves if their care plans state so. Take them along to wherever you are going or if you cannot call another member of staff to stay with them till you get back.
5. Never leave a service user *alone* unattended in the bath when supporting them with personal care.
6. If it's your first time on a service (project), after the induction, make sure you ask for the following information since you may not have enough time to go through all the support plans. Does the service user have major health issues like:

- epilepsy;
- diabetes;
- panic attacks;
- fainting spells;
- asthma?

This should help you assess your potential to work with the intended service user or service users.

7. If you are lone working:
    - keep the main set of keys with you at all times;
    - when leaving the office, always make sure you leave the windows and door locked behind you;
    - keep the portable phone and the mobile phone with you when out of the office;
    - remember to log in with your response team or sister project, stating your starting time and expected finish time;
    - in case of any incident liaise with your response team or the on-call manager or a sister project for support and back-up;
    - in case of an emergency assess the situation and call 999, when the emergency is being dealt with inform the necessary authorities as per the organisation's emergency procedure;
    - document every event as it happened and pass it to the team by documenting a reference in the communication book.
8. Respect the service user living in any given project or a residential care setting as this is their home.
9. Always keep your belongings with you at all times, and if you have medication of any kind where a service user could have access accidentally from your belongings, please hand them over to the line manager or supervisor for safe keeping till the end of your shift.
10. Always sign *in* and *out* of the building at all times.

21.3   Ending the shift

1. Ensure that all entries are completed on daily diaries or log-in book or in the contact sheet of the service users.
2. Ensure that messages are recorded in the communication book, outlining who the message is intended for, dated and signed.
3. Update handover sheet with anything new or any tasks, chores or appointments you were not able to complete during your shift giving the reasons why, e.g. service users unsettled during the entire shift state the nature of the incident
4. Tidy away any work files, filing and leave the office/home/house clean and tidy.
5. Make any notes needed to assist in the handover to incoming staff.
6. Complete a building/security check, walk around and ensure the project is being handed over in a fair clean state.
7. For a smooth and efficient running of handover, it is important that these items are completed accurately and in good time before the next staff come in.
8. Sign off the project

22 Summary: Safety Tips

22.1 Do not perform medical tasks unless you are trained

Examples include:

- giving injections;
- changing dressings, colostomy bags and catheters;
- administering anti-epilepsy emergency drugs like Rectal Diazepam or Buccal Midazolam.

22.2 Follow the organisation's policy and procedure on medication

- Only assist with medications that have been prescribed for service users.
- Follow the medication instructions carefully.
- Store all medications in the medication cabinet and ensure it is locked at all times.

22.3 Use all equipment safely

- Store all equipment in a safe place.
- Make sure it is in good working condition.
- Check equipment before use.
- Report faulty equipment to your manager or supervisor.
- Only use equipment if you have been trained and authorised to do so.
- Wear protective equipment (follow manufacturer's instructions).

22.4 Be prepared for emergencies

- In general you should know the basic emergency first aid and when to call the emergency services. Ask your line manger or shift leader if you have any questions.
- You must report any injuries involving a service user or yourself to your manager or shift leader.

22.5 Report any acts or threats of violence towards you or service users

These include:
- physical or verbal abuse;
- racial or sexual harassment;
- any threats or other behaviour that makes you feel uncomfortable.

22.6 Use caution when travelling away from the project/home

- Always tell someone where you will be, and when you will be back.
- Stay on well-lit paths if walking at night.
- Don't use short cuts.

22.7   Prevent slips, trips and falls

- Keep walkways well lit and free from clutter.
- Use caution and tell others about wet floors or other hazards.
- Make sure carpets are secured.
- Avoid trailing cables across rooms or under carpets.
- Do not stand on a chair or boxes to reach for something. Use stepladder
- Make sure work areas have good lighting.
- Report any dangers.

22.8   Induction workbook

1. How do you prevent slips, trips and falls?

    _____

    _____

2. Why is it important to report any acts or threats of violence towards yourself or a service user?

    _____

    _____

3. Why is it important to follow the organisation's policy and procedure, especially on medication?

    _____

    _____

4. Why is it important for you not to perform medical tasks unless you are trained?

    _____

    _____

5. How would you prepare for emergencies?

    _____

    _____

6. Why is it important to use all equipment safely?

    _____

    _____

Appendix I   List of Acronyms

ABA	Applied Behavioural Analysis
ABC	Antecedent Behaviour Consequences
ACAS	Advisory, Conciliation and Arbitration Service
ADHD	Attention-Deficit Hyperactivity Disorder
AEDs	Anti-Epileptic Drugs
ASD	Autistic Spectrum Disorder(s)
BBD	Body Dysmorphic Disorder
BNF	British National Formulary
BSL	British Sign Language
CARNA	College & Association of Registered Nurses of Alberta
CD	Controlled Drugs
CHRE	Council for Healthcare Regulatory Excellence
CMHTs	Community Mental Health Teams
COSHH	Control of Substances Hazardous to Health
CPS	Complex Partial Seizure
CQC	Care Quality Commission
CSCI	Commission for Social Care Inspection
DBRS	Daily Behaviour Rating Scale
DDA	Disability Discrimination Act
DES	Disability Equality Scheme
DfES	Department for Education and Skills
DoH	Department of Health
DSM-IV	Diagnostic and Statistical Manual of Mental Disorder, 4th Edition
GPs	General Practitioners
GSCC	General Social Care Council
GSL	General Sales List
HACCP	Hazard Analysis and Critical Control Points
HASAWA	Health and Safety at Work Act
HSE	Health and Safety Executive
IT	Information Technology
LD	Learning Disabilities
LOLER	Lifting Operations and Lifting Equipment Regulations
MAR	Medication Administration Record
MDS	Monitored Dosage System
MDT	Multidisciplinary Team
MHA	Mental Health Act
NCSBN	National Council of State Boards of Nursing
NHS	National Health Services
NMS	National Minimum Standards
OCD	Obsessive Compulsive Disorder
P	Pharmacy Medicines

PIDA	Public Interest Disclosure Act
POM	Prescription Only Medication
PPE	Personal Protection Equipment
PRN	Pro Ra Nate
PUWER	Provision and Use of Work Equipment Regulations
QDS	Four Times Daily
RBM	Relation-Based Model
RCD	Residual Current Device
RES	Race Equality Scheme
RIDDOR	Reporting of Injuries, Diseases and Dangerous Occurrences Regulations
RMO	Registered Medical Officer
SALT	Speech and Language Therapist
SPELL	Structure, Positive, Empathy, Low arousal, Links
SPS	Simple Partial Seizure
SWL	Safe Working Load
TD	Twice Daily
TDS	Three Times Daily
WIIIFM	What Is In It For Me?
WRAP	Wellness Recovery Action Planning

Appendix II   Glossary of Terms Used in Bipolar and Other Mental Illness

AMPH (*pronounced Amp*)

Approved Mental Health Practitioner – a social worker or nursing professional who is trained and qualified in the decision to section someone.

CAMHS (*pronounced Cams*)

Child and Adolescent Mental Health for those under 18 years of age

Care plan

List of action points decided upon and written down by the person with bipolar and their support team for the future

CPA

Care Plan Approach – a care plan which is regularly reviewed with the care coordinator and others involved in the person's care, which includes risk assessment, needs met and unmet. It is also used when someone is being discharged from hospital to ease their transition back to their life outside.

CPN

Community Psychiatric Nurse – nurses who support those people with mental illnesses when they are not in hospital either from their homes or in supported accommodation

Crisis team

The crisis team offer out-of hours support or more intensive support; it varies on where the person lives

Cyclothymia

Where depressive and maniac symptoms lasts for two years or more but are not serious enough for diagnosis of bipolar disorder

dual diagnosis

Where a diagnosis such as bipolar disorder is accompanied by another condition such as alcoholism

hallucination

A a perception of something not real; can be visual, auditory – can be voices but also other sounds, tactile, smell and taste

hypomania

A persistent, mild elevation of mood

hypothyroidism

A condition where the thyroid gland does not produce enough of the hormone thyroxine – it can be caused by taking Lithium, a drug used to treat bipolar disorder

Independent Mental Health Advocacy   The role of independent mental health advocates http://www.nmhdu.org.uk

Informal patient

Someone who agrees to admission to a psychiatric hospital

Mania

An unnaturally high euphoric mood

Manic depression

Another name for bipolar disorder, less often used today

Mixed state/episode

Where symptoms of mania and depression occur at the same time

NICE	National Institute for Clinical Excellence – an independent organisation responsible for providing national guidance on the promotion of good health and the prevention and treatment of ill health in the UK
PALS	Patients Advice and Liaison Services
Paranoia	Delusions of persecution and belief of a perceived threat towards oneself
Psychiatrist	A person qualified in the study and treatment of mental illnesses
Psychologist	A person qualified in the study of the human mind and its functions
Psychosis	A loss of contact with external reality includes paranoia, delusions of grandeur and hallucinations. Does not describe someone who is dangerous
Rapid cycle	Experiencing more than four mood swings in one year
Sectioned	A compulsory admittance to a psychiatric hospital under the Mental Health Act
Service user	Someone who receives mental health services
Ultra rapid cycling	Experiencing monthly, weekly, daily or hourly mood swings
Unipolar	A word used to describe depression where only low moods are experienced, without the high moods also experienced by those with bipolar disorder. It is quite common to receive a wrong diagnosis of unipolar disorder before a correct diagnosis of bipolar disorder
Voluntary patient	Someone who has agreed to admittance to a psychiatric hospital

Index

Note: page numbers in italic refer to illustrations.

Lightning Source UK Ltd.
Milton Keynes UK
UKOW06f1917240215

246836UK00004B/242/P